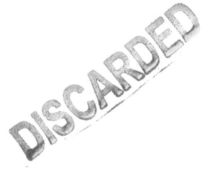

The
Therapy
Sourcebook

Francine M. Roberts, Psy.D., R.N.

LOWELL HOUSE
Los Angeles
CONTEMPORARY BOOKS
Chicago

Disclaimer: The clients described in this manuscript are disguised composites. Resemblance to any real person or situation is not intended. Descriptions are fiction, using altered details and names, and aspects of many people gathered into one, for the purpose of illustration.

Library of Congress Cataloging-in-Publication Data

Roberts, Francine M.
    The therapy sourcebook / Francine M. Roberts.
      p. cm.
    Includes bibliographical references and index.
    ISBN 1-56565-793-4
    1. Psychotherapy—Popular works. 2. Mental illness. I. Title.
RC480.515.R6   1997   97-45880
616.89′14—dc21   CIP

Requests for such permissions should be addressed to:
Lowell House
2020 Avenue of the Stars, Suite 300
Los Angeles, California 90067

Lowell House books can be purchased at special discounts when ordered in bulk for premiums and special sales.

Publisher: Jack Artenstein
Associate Publisher, Lowell House Adult: Bud Sperry
Director of Publishing Services: Rena Copperman
Managing Editor: Maria Magallanes
Text Design: Cheryl Carrington

Illustrations: LifeART Images. Copyright © 1989–1997 by TechPool Studios, Inc., USA (p. 60, 62)

Manufactured in the United States of America
10 9 8 7 6 5 4 3 2 1

Contents

Acknowledgments

I wish to thank the following people for their support and encouragement during the completion of this manuscript: Maureen Mitchell, for telling me I could write; Mervyn Mitchell, for his belief in me and his careful and considered contributions to the manuscript. To Zoltan and Shirley Roberts, for their interest and feedback. To William Stuart Mitchell and Dr. Barry Bricklin, for taking time to read drafts and contributing perspectives that are decidedly different from my own. To my colleagues, Mary Ellen Santucci and Joan Dresh, who take publication in stride, as just another part of the job. To my husband and best friend, Eric, for his limitless emotional and technical support. To the teachers along the way who have provided a comprehensive education. And to the patients who have allowed me to witness their transformations.

Introduction

I am writing this book because psychotherapy works. Talking helps. Therapy offers a vast array of techniques designed to promote positive change. We all want to be happy. When something interferes with our happiness, we look for ways to alter the situation. Therapy can be an amazing journey that results in transformation, development, and healing. Psychotherapy is a proven method for enhancing how we feel and function, as complex bio-psycho-social-spiritual beings. For some people, it is life enriching; for others, lifesaving. For most people who experience it, psychotherapy is a deeply meaningful process that produces satisfactory results.

Psychotherapy evolved, in part because of a natural curiosity about the mind and an innate tendency to strive for our highest potential. When we have symptoms, we want to fix them. Because we are capable of self-observation, we are destined to wonder about the dance and play of the mind. We want to understand how the mind works. If we can understand our psychology, we can influence it.

Given ideal circumstances, and a supportive environment, we might progress through life with little difficulty. We could establish an accurate sense of self and a positive outlook about the future. We would trust ourselves and others. We would be easily able to meet the challenges that arise in our lives. However, few of us live in ideal circumstances. Ordinary life presents challenges and disappointments. *Normal* development can result in uncomfortable conflicts and maturational crises. The times in which we live present cultural, political, or personal situations that can become traumatic. As individuals, we seek methods for achieving a resolution to these issues. As a culture, we are interested in promoting interpersonal growth, relief of distress, and the pursuit of happiness. Psychotherapy offers a method for personal growth, symptom relief, and self-actualization.

My inspiration for writing comes from the successes I see being achieved, every day, in therapy. I have seen people grow as a result of self-exploration and make changes subsequent to recognizing ineffective patterns of coping. Through therapy, many people are able to clarify problems, implement changes, and relinquish ineffective behaviors. These successes are a testament to the power of the human mind, as well as evidence of the human spirit.

We all experience some level of psychological distress. Through these challenges, we can understand something of what it is like for people who have severe symptoms. When we see someone else in distress, we are reminded of our own challenges. Because we can have this perspective, and be aware of the similarities, we develop compassion. We can be sensitive to the needs of people who have trouble adapting to the demands of everyday life. We understand wanting to be free from symptoms of distress. We understand the urgent need for effective interventions. Psychotherapy is a method for reducing psychological symptoms and correcting the conditions that maintain maladaptive behavior patterns.

Sometimes, people will take the work of just a few sessions in therapy and use what is achieved throughout their lifetime. For some people, gains are small. But at times, change can be monumental. It has been said that therapy can transform misery into common, ordinary unhappiness. On the surface, this may seem like a minor change. However, when translated into real-life experience, this is really quite an accomplishment! My experience has been that therapy can offer a resolution to misery and much, much more. Participating in therapy can be an enriching, validating, and self-affirming experience.

As a practicing psychotherapist, I am always searching for methods and theories that will be helpful in alleviating emotional distress and promoting personal growth. Psychotherapy is a blend of art and science, of faith and fact, and of intellect and relationship. Psychotherapy is an art because it uses creativity and expression. It is a science because it is based on more than a century of worldwide research. The sciences of psychology and psychiatry offer facts gained from research as evidence to support their theories. Therapy requires some faith in the process and in the promise of growth and change. Therapy involves an intellectual understanding that develops within the context of a unique relationship. Therapy is a dynamic, evolving process that focuses on change, growth, and understanding.

Each person's experience in therapy will be different. People seek therapy for all sorts of reasons, with many different expectations, and receive many different forms of treatment. For example, one person might need therapy for mild symptoms of depression, and choose to work with a cognitive psychotherapist. Therapy might last for ten sessions every other week, and use lots of homework exercises. Another person might go into psychoanalysis to understand relationship difficulties. They might meet four times a week for four, five, or even ten years. Sessions would involve free association, exploring the unconscious, and resolving underlying conflicts. Another person might go to a psychiatrist for anxiety, and after an evaluation, decide to use medications to relieve symptoms. They might meet once every two months for fifteen minutes to review the impact of pharmacological treatments. Still another person might go for psychotherapy and use hypnosis to conquer their fears and anxieties. Some people go alone for therapy, others meet in families or groups. Information in this book is presented in a way that attempts to recognize and respect the unique form and character of each therapy experience.

If you ask twelve psychotherapists the same question, you will undoubtedly get twelve different answers. Every theory has some value. When I say anxiety is a result of conflicting forces within the mind, biological theorists will disagree vehemently, and insist that anxiety is a neurochemical, genetically determined reaction related to the neurotransmitter gamma-aminobutyric acid (GABA). Behaviorists see it differently from analysts, and analysts see it differently from biological psychologists. Rather than seeing different perspectives as competing, they can be seen as complementary. What is more likely true is that each perspective helps to explain some part of our complex human experience. Understanding mental functioning requires biological, psychological, behavioral, molecular, sociological, environmental, and developmental perspectives. Our work is to study and evaluate the variety of perspectives, then work with the ideas that most aptly fit the specific issue.

The Promise of Psychotherapy

Psychotherapy is safe and effective. It can help you find more effective ways to cope rather than use methods that are futile or uncomfortable. Therapy can heighten your awareness and offer techniques for changing behaviors. The process of psychotherapy can offer new ways of thinking about life's challenges and foster the development of innovative problem-solving approaches. Therapy is a method for quickening personal development, as well as for solving problems. It offers a dynamic opportunity for personal growth. The therapy process can provide insights that clarify the meaning and purpose of our lives and help us avoid responses that are painful or pointless. This book is an invitation to explore the world of psychotherapy.

Psychotherapy is not a panacea. It cannot help everyone, all the time. However, when a genuine effort is made by both the therapist and client, positive effects are likely to occur. Depending on the amount of time and effort devoted to therapy, goals might include changing selected behaviors or developing an understanding of patterns in your relationships. You might want to understand better your own thinking or feelings. You may choose to explore what conscious and unconscious influences have an impact on your mental well-being. You might explore different perspectives or ways to think about problems. You might try new behaviors, with experiential exercises. Your relationship with a therapist can add a unique component to your interpersonal history. The therapist may become one of the internal mental images you rely on for support and guidance. Therapy will become what you make of it. Your individual goals and personal style will determine the exact nature of the therapeutic work you choose.

Thinking of Therapy?

You do not need to be *sick* or *abnormal* to enter psychotherapy. In fact, it is often the healthiest person in a system who comes for therapy first. Therapy can be beneficial if you are interested in learning more about yourself, changing behaviors that don't work, or finding new perspectives in relationships.

Perhaps you are curious to read this book because you are considering therapy. Or, someone you know may need help. Most people consider therapy when they are having problems they cannot solve themselves. Questions about psychotherapy often arise when someone is struggling with uncomfortable emotions or worrisome inner conflicts. Stress at work or at home may prompt you to look for a therapist. Conflicts in relationships may appear overwhelming. Feelings of loneliness, frustration, or confusion may interfere with achieving your goals and desired satisfaction. You may be noticing patterns of behavior that don't produce desired results, such as frequent arguments or compulsive behaviors. You may be aware of feelings that are uncomfortable or un-pleasant moods that linger. Or you may have vague feelings of *dis*-ease and diffuses anxieties. Any concern that persists over time and begins to interfere with achieving life's full potential is a valid reason for seeking a psychotherapy consultation.

You might begin by asking yourself, "What are my goals?" Start by clarifying what symptoms or issues you would like to address. You do not need to have a clear idea about what your *exact* focus will be before beginning, but identifying a general purpose for the consultation may be helpful. For example, you might decide to talk with someone about relationship issues or work stresses. You might want to develop some effective stress-management skills. If you are experiencing distress that does not seem to be improving with your current efforts, you may wish to investigate the benefits that psychotherapy might offer.

Most people who are considering therapy talk it over with someone who is close to them. You might ask friends about their experiences with therapy. You might speak informally to a therapist you know. You could even call several therapists to discuss your concerns briefly over the phone and whether a consultation should be scheduled. Most therapists will be eager to meet for an evaluation and to discuss whether you should start an ongoing treatment.

You may wish to learn as much as you can from sources whom you trust as you make a decision about whether or not to investigate therapy for yourself. A great deal of information about psychology, mental health, and treatment is easily available through publications, the Internet, and broadcast media. Some of what you find will resonate with your instincts about your concerns or goals. What you find may seem to match comfortably your own understanding. Other information will be less useful or may seem inaccurate. When contradictory information is encountered, evaluate it carefully, with an open mind. Perhaps it is simply a new perspective. Or, the alternative perspective may not be helpful and ought to be discarded.

When you begin to consider therapy, it is generally because you feel a pressing need for some change or personal development. In that case, your journey has already begun! Take heart that therapists are eager and available to facilitate your progress. What you encounter along your journey will be evaluated for meaningfulness, and through persistent efforts in psychotherapy, your desires can often be achieved. Therapy is an exciting process. Learning about the mind and human behavior can be a lifelong pursuit. Therapy can help you expand the range of coping options available and support you in meeting life's challenges. I urge you to value yourself enough to take the time to know yourself and to more fully experience who you really are through psychotherapy.

My Background

I have been privileged to collaborate with many clients in diverse settings with complex problems and watch their positive transformations. I began my clinical career in an urban university hospital, working with people experiencing physical health problems. In helping clients with medical conditions cope with treatments and surgery, I learned firsthand what a profound impact psychological adaptation can have on physical recovery. I was delighted to discover that the simple act of listening to clients talk about their illness experiences had marked, positive effects.

I wanted to learn more about how the brain functioned and how physiological functioning was integrated with psychological processes. I began to work with clients with severe mental illness in an inpatient setting, and saw how profoundly disturbed psychosocial functioning can become. I worked with clients from all walks of life who were experiencing serious symptoms that resulted in difficulty adapting to the demands of daily living. In learning about these severe disorders it became clear that social, community, and economic conditions can have a significant effect on the quality of life for someone with altered psychological functioning.

During graduate school, I had experiences working with children, adolescents, and highly capable adult clients. I had opportunities to work with clients with less severe disorders and whose focus in treatment was on achieving their full potential. Through the talents of skilled mentors and supervisors, I began to learn the craft of psychotherapy.

I was invited to a state-run psychiatric hospital for clients with severe, chronic mental illness. I learned about the damages that can occur with a lifetime of institutionalization, as well as the risks faced by clients with disabilities who attempt to survive in the community. These clients helped me remember how the simple aspects of life, such as sharing a cup of coffee, or breathing the morning fresh air can be so valuable. This was a select segment of society that had adjusted to schizophrenia, and I saw how clients who were psychologically challenged could comfortably adapt in a setting that understands and tolerates their idiosyncratic behaviors.

I spent time working in a major metropolitan psychiatric emergency center. Here we evaluated and stabilized clients in psychological crises. I have seen thousands of patients, individually and in groups. Some encounters were brief and lasted a few hours. Other interactions have been more intense and lasted for years. The range of adaptation in this diverse group of clients gave me an appreciation for how varied life experience can be. I have been able to observe talented clinicians, dedicated to the well-being of their clients, implementing the full gamut of treatment options.

Since becoming a licensed psychologist, I have worked in the community with geriatric clients and provided outpatient psychotherapy services in a managed-care setting. Currently, I work as an assistant professor at Thomas Jefferson University in Philadelphia and have a private practice in clinical psychology.

A Word About Titles

There has been a great debate about what to call people who come for psychotherapy consultation. We have struggled with titles in an attempt to reduce the stigma associated with seeking treatment. In the early years, people who came for treatment were called "patients" because most of the treatment was provided by medical doctors. Later, as therapy became more widely applied, we saw that people who went for consultation were not necessarily ill, and we adopted the term "client." The current term preferred in some circles is "consumer," which emphasizes that people who come for therapy are purchasing a service. It is not accurate to say that all people who seek treatment are sick, and thus are patients. I think that consumer is a cumbersome title that minimizes the importance of the treatment relationship. Because of when and where I was trained, I generally refer to people who come for therapy as clients. I believe this most accurately reflects an equal relationship and better reflects the nature of the collaborative process. My intention is to convey respect and an egalitarian arrangement between participants in therapy. I believe we are truly partners.

The Therapy Sourcebook

You may wish to use this book as a springboard for action. If you are interested in exploring the process of psychotherapy, learning some new skills, developing some new perspectives, or making some changes, you can use this book as a guide. Schedule an evaluation with a therapist who can explore the potential benefits of treatment in your particular situation. This book encourages you to experience psychotherapy for yourself and see where the dialogue may lead you.

If you are considering consultation with a therapist, it may be helpful to learn as much as you can about the process. The information contained in *The Therapy Sourcebook* may be used to stimulate a dialogue with family members, friends, and professional counselors. Learn about the types of therapy available and methods of treatment that may be most helpful. It may be beneficial to interview several clinicians before selecting a therapist. It is important to find someone who is compatible with your style and thinking. *The Therapy Sourcebook* can assist you in making informed choices. Therapists may wish to use it to orient clients to options, techniques, and approaches in treatment.

The Therapy Sourcebook is a guide to understanding therapy. If you have little or no experience with psychotherapy, it is comprehensive and easy to understand. In addition, there is information for the therapy-wise consumer. This book is designed to assist you with any questions you have about therapy. *The Therapy Sourcebook* addresses a broad range of information about mental health and mental health treatment. However, each subject can be understood in greater depth.

Resources for finding more complete information will be included.

This book is not intended to be a substitute for consultation with a qualified mental health provider. It in no way implies a treatment relationship between the author and reader. You need to evaluate the information presented and incorporate what fits and discard what doesn't apply. This book is simply a source of information about therapy. Perhaps the best way to use it is in collaboration with a therapist. You might review pertinent sections together, discuss options, and develop a plan that will help you reach your particular goals.

Every attempt has been made to present information without bias, as well as give equal consideration to diverse points of view. Every clinician develops beliefs about mental health and treatment based on study and experience. These biases inevitably affect the theories and interventions adopted and utilized by each clinician. You may disagree with some of what is presented. The therapist you consult may have different ideas and perspectives. I encourage you to evaluate ideas from a variety of perspectives and develop a broad understanding of the mind and psychotherapy.

Those of you reading undoubtedly come from varying levels of experience with psychotherapy. Readers may be participants who sit on either side of the couch. Some of you may have years of experience and study, while others are relative newcomers to the process. Some of you may be clinicians; many of you are clients. When you are reading this book, you must evaluate how the offered ideas fit with your developing understanding and experience.

The Therapy Sourcebook begins with an overview of psychotherapy and a review of mental health and mental illness. A brief presentation of theories of mental health, personality development, and emotions will be offered. A discussion of major diagnostic categories is included. The next two chapters provide an overview of therapy and how to get started. Subsequent sections explore different forms of therapy. Sections are included to make you familiar with behavioral, cognitive, biological, and psychodynamic therapies. A discussion of aspects of life that are naturally therapeutic is included. Chapters on children, termination, resources, and becoming a therapist are also offered.

CHAPTER 1

Therapy: An Overview

What Is Psychotherapy?

Therapy is a method for understanding why you do, what you do, and for influencing how you respond to life's challenges. Psychotherapy involves a systematic approach to making changes. At its heart, psychotherapy is an interpersonal collaboration, a relationship, designed to relieve distress and promote optimal development. It applies scientific methods to alleviate symptoms and facilitate adaptation. The process of therapy may involve exploring the layers of the mind or analyzing behavioral patterns. Sometimes it is an active, problem-solving process. At other times it may be quiet and introspective. Psychotherapy may involve talking about concerns, with a goal of finding solutions to conflicts and understanding behavior. It might involve exercises and prescribed experiences.

Anyone can choose to go into therapy. It is a process that welcomes all who are interested. For the client, there are no prerequisites of skill, insight, or knowledge. The client brings a problem and a willingness to collaborate on a solution. The therapist brings expert knowledge and systematic attention to the client. The therapist may assist through nondirective, consistent support or offer active suggestions about behavioral choices and identify consequences to chosen actions. The therapist, and the process, will adapt to your style, level of ability, and unique areas of concern.

Jerome Frank (1963), a professor of psychiatry at Johns Hopkins University, describes psychotherapy in his book *Persuasion and Healing* as a type of "influence" that involves a healer and a client who meet in structured and formal contacts. The therapist has an expertise in the methods of change and an understanding of human functioning. The client is anyone who seeks relief and believes that the healer can provide it. The healer is granted rights to practice treatment because of his education and role in society. A structured series of meetings is designed to produce emotional, behavioral, or attitudinal changes. The therapist uses his influence to facilitate adaptation, acceptance, and change.

Therapy offers a setting where you can be honest with yourself. In most of our relationships, we have obligations and role expectations. Meeting these expectations may interfere with an open expression of what we think or how we really feel in a particular situation. Therapy provides the opportunity to self-examine aspects that might seem unacceptable to express in other places. Therapy can offer an opportunity for regular, structured self-exploration. When a regular meeting is scheduled each week, you know you will focus on yourself during this time. Because an appointment is scheduled ahead of time, introspection, self-study, or behavioral change cannot be postponed indefinitely. In many ways, this may provide a sense of security. You may feel freer to concentrate on other matters, knowing that for at least one hour a week there will be time to focus on your personal concerns. If you are reluctant to address some issue, a regularly scheduled appointment may provide an inescapable opportunity for introspection.

The assurance of privacy and an atmosphere of acceptance make it possible to examine parts of ourselves that we are ashamed of or embarrassed by. We can open our closet doors, and with the help of a skilled, supportive therapist allow our skeletons to come out. One psychology professor reminds students that most people live in terror of opening these closet doors, building the skeletons in our minds into ominous monsters. When the door is finally opened, we discover the skeleton has long ago turned to dust, and its power to terrorize us is disintegrated. Some therapists have suggested that therapy requires "rigorous honesty." True progress can be made when we are able to admit to ourselves, and to another human being, our limitations and shortcomings. We begin to make changes when we admit that there is something wrong.

Psychotherapy can also be a place for learning new skills, such as self-hypnosis or visualization. Through these techniques we can influence thoughts and images that may operate below our conscious awareness, but which can exert a profound effect on our well-being. Psychotherapy is a safe and effective way to alter the mind-body system to facilitate more adaptive responses.

Therapy allows for the clarification and identification of emotions. This is perhaps one of the most helpful aspects of a dynamic therapy. Often our emotions are confusing, hard to identify, and at times may be overwhelming. Therapy can assist you to identify and cope with feelings. Identifying what we are feeling allows us to be able to respond more effectively to our emotions. As emotional experiences are explored, feelings and perceptions can be validated. Confidence in the accuracy of our perceptions grows, and increasingly we can trust our personal interpretations.

Therapy is an investment in yourself and an affirmation of your worth. As the therapist listens and understands the client's experiences, the client feels less alone. The therapist can validate feelings and perceptions, which promotes an increased sense of personal identity. When the therapist can genuinely say, "It is understandable that you would feel that way," or "I see it just as you do," the client often experiences a sense of relief. Guilt about feelings of anger or shame about impulses can be alleviated. The client can be reassured that their perceptions are indeed valid, and discrepancies between feelings and intellectual conceptions can be reconciled.

For example, one client described witnessing as a child terrible arguments between his parents. The father suffered from severe emotional difficulties and when arguing would become violent and destructive toward the furniture. Even though the client was sent to his bedroom during these fights, he witnessed his parents breaking chairs and tables by sneaking out to the top of the stairs and watching below. The family kept a set of spare furniture in the garage, and after these episodes they would replace the broken furniture with intact pieces. The broken pieces were taken to the garage, and the father developed a hobby of repairing furniture in his spare time. When the client awoke in the morning, his parents denied that an argument had occurred. New furniture was in place. Although he had witnessed it the night before, his parents acted as if nothing had happened. The client developed difficulty trusting his own perceptions. It was difficult for him to assess accurately when conflict was occurring in his current relationships. He had particular difficulty understanding the behaviors he witnessed during childhood in relation to conflict resolution. He would notice vague feelings of anger in his gut but deny its occurrence intellectually. This pattern developed because of a denial of his sensory perceptions as a child. The client stopped trusting what he observed and had a tendency to focus selectively in situations involving conflict, denying any destructive effects. Through therapy, the client was better able to recognize aggressive aspects of conflict and to identify emotions as they occurred during disagreements. The therapist was able to validate the client's perceptions, resulting in his increasing ability to trust his perceptions, particularly in situations of conflict.

Psychotherapy may appear to be a conversation, and in

some forms, it is. However, it is not an ordinary conversation. Although the interaction may appear to be casual, when a therapist is working, words are carefully chosen. The skilled therapist is aware that communications are interventions and must be considered carefully before they are offered. As the therapist listens and communicates, he carefully evaluates the client's response to verbal and nonverbal exchanges. For example, in response to a statement that is intended to provide support or encourage clarification, the therapist would expect to see the client relax and feel more comfortable opening up about an issue. The therapist monitors the impact of chosen words and guides the interaction in a way that facilitates achieving the goals of treatment.

Even the greeting at the beginning of each session can have an impact on the therapeutic environment. One client in therapy noted that when she says, "Hi! How are you doing?" as a greeting at the door, the therapist always replies, "Good afternoon" or "Good morning." Never, "I'm fine. How are you?" The client was curious about this consistent discrepancy in communication. The therapist is using a model of therapy that attempts to minimize her personal impact and limit the focus on the therapist. Her carefully chosen words help to establish an environment that focuses attention on the client's well-being, not her own. The goal of the therapy is ultimately the client's self-exploration, not exploration of the therapist's well-being. The therapist's greeting is designed to set a tone that encourages the client to focus on her own functioning.

An exchange of energy occurs in therapy. As the therapist and client develop their relationship, energy flows between participants. There may be excitement or anxiety as the collaboration develops. The therapy relationship changes both participants and contributes to personal growth in the therapist as well as in the client. It may be readily apparent that the client is taking support from the therapist's energy, but the therapist may also take energy from the client. It can be energizing to witness the development and progress of a fellow human being. Often, the therapist feels renewed from the collaborative process and takes energy in the form of increased interest for the work. It is exciting to see others grow into their full potential, as well as learn about human potential through a collaborative relationship that heightens conscious awareness.

Psychotherapy contains an inherent risk of change. Many clients make an appointment with a therapist because of a conscious desire for change. However, when the opportunity for change is at hand, clients often feel ambivalent. Some people unconsciously begin to mobilize defenses that resist change. No matter how uncomfortable our pain, it is familiar. Familiar pain can at times be preferable to the unknown possibilities of change.

In addition, the act of asking for help implies an acknowledgment that something is wrong. It can be difficult to admit that there is a problem and even harder to admit that we may play a role in its continuation. We may feel guilty about symptoms. Needing help may reinforce feelings of self-blame. Some people fear that asking for counseling indicates that they are "crazy." Most people who enter therapy reach a point of distress, where the potential benefits of change outweigh the fears of asking for help. When the pain we are experiencing outweighs the embarrassment of recognizing a problem, we begin to look for a therapist.

The Process of Psychotherapy

Most people have a sense of relief when they make that first appointment for consultation. You may feel that although there is some problem, at least now you are taking a positive step toward a solution. Once a therapeutic alliance has been established and a therapist is selected, most people feel a sense of support. The very act of entering therapy places you in a partnership, which is designed to improve current difficulties. Early meetings in therapy can be used for establishing a trusting relationship.

A unique relationship is formed in each collaboration. You and your therapist will create the therapy together. Together, the therapist and client evolve a process of change that is dynamic and highly personalized. The client with emotional distress is faced with the seemingly enormous task of finding a skilled and competent clinician who works in a manner that is consistent with their own thinking. If a therapist and client are incompatible, generally the client will dismiss the process as unhelpful and discontinue treatment or seek help from someone else.

Positive feelings in therapy are beneficial and facilitate exploration and problem solving. Believing in the overall effectiveness of the process can help to sustain the work when it evokes challenging feelings or concerns. You should have a strong sense of working together with your therapist on issues, as well as feeling supported. Viewing your therapist as an ally and advocate can ease difficult challenges when they arise. Perhaps it is inevitable that in any dynamic therapy relationship, feelings of fear, anger, and disappointment will emerge. Sometimes, the therapy experience is pleasant and comforting. However, change and exploration can become a tumultuous process. As you become aware of negative or shameful feelings therapy may produce anxiety. Psychotherapy offers opportunities embedded in these crises of change. Although therapy cannot change personal history, it can change our reactions to previous events. We can develop new ways to respond to events in our lives. In therapy, it is possible to learn new ways to think, and experience new aspects of emotion and behavior.

You may wish to develop a treatment plan in collaboration with your therapist. Be specific about your goals. Goals may involve symptom removal; to stop vomiting after meals, to stop compulsively checking the stove or washing your hands, or to decrease angry outbursts. Goals may involve resolving conflicts or developing new skills, for example, resolution of depression and anger, feelings of loss or grief, or improving problem solving, or capacity for emotion.

What Psychotherapy Is Not

Psychotherapy is not a guaranteed process. No on can predetermine results. It is the result of a unique interaction that will produce unique results. Results will vary depending on the match between the types of problems encountered and the resources available to work toward a solution. If the client brings a serious difficulty to treatment and neither the therapist nor the client has sufficient coping resources, positive progress might be slow and gains limited. However, when concerns are of a more limited nature and the client and the therapist are able to identify easily resources that can bolster coping efforts, results of therapy are more likely to be satisfactory.

Therapy is not mind control. Changes and choices that you make are done so with a free will. The therapist may have an influence on your thinking and can offer alternative perspectives to your own. But the choices about what elements of the process you incorporate into your thinking or daily actions is ultimately your own. An ethical therapist will not bully or coerce patients into types of thought or actions. An ethical therapist will encourage you to evaluate alternatives and support your autonomous choices. Although therapy is by nature an interdependent relationship, ultimately the therapist strives to be obsolete and to have the client function with added autonomy. Most legitimate forms of therapy discourage excessive dependence on the therapist or therapy, recognizing that it is better for clients to use their own resources toward independence.

Psychotherapy is not necessarily quick. It takes time to

make an accurate assessment of symptoms and situations. Implementing change takes time; developing insight has its own unique pace. Symptoms and problems take time to develop, and so do solutions. Although shifting reimbursement patterns have shortened the duration of most treatment, the process of change will proceed with its own schedule. It may be necessary to work with information gained in one or two sessions, over time, evaluating for yourself how these ideas might be used in everyday life. An important aspect of effective therapy is the readiness for change. When interventions coincide with a readiness to make changes, work in sessions may have a more significant impact. Progress might also hit plateaus and seem to stall for a period of time. Keep in mind that the human experience is intricate and complex, and developing solutions may take time.

Although some forms of psychotherapy involve bodywork, such as bioenergetics and rolfing, psychotherapy generally does not involve touching. Although there is no denying that touch can be beneficial in some contexts (for example, in a massage, hugs from family or friends, or in intimate relationships), most forms of psychotherapy do not involve physical contact. *Sexual* contact is never acceptable in psychotherapy. I am suspicious of therapists who feel compelled to hug their clients. They are usually poorly trained and ineffectual. Sexual contact with clients is prohibited, and in most circumstances, illegal. Sexual contact is a violation of professional ethical standards and grounds for loss of licensed privileges. If you are approached by a therapist in a sexual manner, confront the therapist, then report the incident to the state and national licensing boards.

Therapy is not mind reading; you must tell the therapist what is on your mind. Psychotherapy is not fortune-telling, predicting the future, nor dialoguing with deceased spirits. Therapists may be many things, but in general they are not clairvoyant. As a rule, therapists do not possess extrasensory perceptions. Therapy does not involve communicating with the dead or channeling beings without bodies. All of these activities may be entertaining, beneficial, or life-enriching, but they are not to be confused with professional psychotherapy.

What's in It for Me?

You might be wondering, "Why should I go into psychotherapy? What benefits will I get?" First, and perhaps most important, you will get direct support. Before initiating a consultation, clients are often struggling alone with an issue. By definition, consulting a therapist gives you an additional person to focus with you on the problem. The therapist brings energy reserves to the problem and can bolster a depleted system by supporting various elements of the dynamic situation.

The therapist provides a fresh perspective. He may see things differently and offer interpretations of situations and clarification of emotions. He might introduce new ways to think or act. The therapist can offer a perspective based on years of study of the human experience and the benefits of many hours spent working to help people change.

The therapist can provide renewed hope and the experience of working with many situations that the client feels are hopeless or overwhelming. For example, the client may feel overwhelmed by anxiety, only to discover that the techniques offered by the therapist can be immediately effective in reducing stress. A client has often exhausted many coping resources before consulting a therapist. The therapist has learned methods of working with severe difficulties that will enhance the chances for successful coping.

Types of Psychotherapy

Individual psychotherapy involves a therapist and a client meeting regularly. It allows for maximum privacy and disclosure, and concentrated feedback from the therapist. Couples therapy can be used to work effectively on relationship issues. This involves a therapist working with a couple as a client, meeting together and/or individually, with the goal of strengthening the relationship. Family therapy involves one or two therapists meeting with members of a family in a variety of combinations. Group therapy involves a group of unrelated individuals meeting with one or two therapists, with a focus on members' concerns and interpersonal relationships. Group therapy is particularly useful for clients with common issues.

Who Can Provide Psychotherapy?

The practice of psychotherapy is restricted to those qualified by licensing regulations. This includes a psychologist, psychiatrist, social worker, or advanced practice nurse. Each of these disciplines offers training for clinical practice. A psychologist has a doctoral degree that focuses on mental functioning and research. A psychiatrist has a doctorate in medicine and post-doctoral training in mental health. A social worker has a master's or doctoral degree, with an education that focuses on psychosocial and system functioning. An advanced practice nurse has a master's or doctoral degree, with a focus on holistic functioning.

Therapists are educated and trained clinically in a number of respected theoretical traditions. Psychologists are trained in some combination of behavioral, biological, and psychodynamic theories of the mind. Psychiatrists come from a medical, behavioral, and psychodynamic perspective. Social workers study systems theory and relationships, as well as other approaches. The major theories include: biological/medical; psychodynamic/psychoanalytic; behavioral/learning theory; cognitive; and existential/humanistic perspectives. A skilled clinical practitioner will be able to incorporate ideas from all these theories, but he will usually be highly skilled in one or two areas. The therapist selects the most appropriate approach for the specific client, in a specific situation. If the therapist believes that the client can benefit from an approach they do not themselves practice, a referral to a colleague should be made.

Within these disciplines, each training program and each clinician adopts a theoretical framework. Most clinicians, when questioned, will describe themselves as eclectic, meaning they blend the major theories. More accurately, a well-trained clinician will understand all the major theories and, although he will have a preference for one or two, he will use other theories as warranted given the situation and the client. For example, I work with primarily a psychodynamic approach. This means that when a client is able, we will attempt to discover and resolve unconscious conflicts that result in dysfunction. However, I have also used relaxation training, a behavioral technique, to treat job-performance anxiety. I occasionally consult with a psychiatrist who will prescribe medications for selected clients. Although it is not my preference, if a client is predisposed to focusing on thoughts, I will use a cognitive approach to correct thinking distortions.

In addition to education and supervised clinical experiences, in order to practice psychotherapy, the state board of occupational affairs must grant a license to practice. This usually requires evidence of good character (or at least no evidence to the contrary, such as a felony conviction); a number of supervised practice hours; endorsement from qualified practitioners in the field; and passing a competency exam, both national and local. Obtaining a license to practice does not allow the clinician to provide any and all services defined in the practice of said profession. The therapist must be able to demonstrate competence to provide that service, specifically didactic and experiential training in that service. This means that although a license to practice psychology includes treating children, a therapist can only see children if they have had special classes and the opportunity for supervised work with children. Clinicians have a legal responsibility to maintain competence in their area of practice through consultation and continuing education.

Can We Be Friends?

In some ways, the therapy relationship resembles a friendship. It involves two people who meet regularly to talk about feelings and experiences. The therapist and client often develop feelings of mutual respect and fondness. There is a mutual interest in maintaining an ongoing interaction and in fostering increasing intimacy. Although these elements are common in both social and therapeutic relationships, there are significant differences between these two types of relationships.

The purpose of the therapy relationship is to address the client's needs. Although it is certain that both the client and the therapist often benefit from interactions, the focus and function of the interactions is to foster the development of the client's well-being. Friendship generally involves a mutual beneficial exchange, with an equal focus on both participants' needs. The therapy relationship is limited by time and place. The client does not have random or continuous access to the therapist. Meetings can only take place at scheduled times.

Therapeutic relationships are structured by clinical theories and provide specific interventions designed to promote the client's growth and development. Friends may be able to listen and lend support, but there is no organizing framework that guides interactions. A therapist can have greater objectivity because she has no stake in the outcome of your life choices except to hope for your optimal adjustment. Although friends may be relatively neutral, in general they have some position at stake when giving you advice.

Therapists are bound by an ethical mandate to avoid dual relationships. For this reason, clients and therapists should not also be friends. Even after therapy has ended, the relationship is a professional one. Likewise, if you are friends with someone who happens to also practice psychotherapy, a treatment relationship should not be established. Even though elements of friendship may be present, professional obligations supercede social interests.

Fees

Typical charges for a single therapy session range from seventy to one hundred and thirty dollars per visit. Social workers tend to charge lower fees, with an average of seventy to one hundred dollars a visit. Psychologists range from eighty to one hundred and ten dollars per visit. Psychiatrists fees may be slightly higher and range from ninety to one hundred and thirty dollars a visit. Fees for evaluations might be slightly higher. Fees for medication management may be lower but involve shorter appointments.

Some therapists set fees that are absolute. Insurance companies require set fees that do not vary. Be prepared to find that insurance does not reimburse generously for mental health treatment. If you decide to pursue ongoing treatment, it might be helpful to plan to put part of your income away for regular therapy expenses. It is essential to find a therapist who is willing to offer treatment within your budget. Therapy must be affordable in order for you to participate over time. When you are paying for treatment out of pocket, you have more flexibility in choosing the therapist and determining how long treatment may continue. Some therapists work on a sliding-fee scale. They offer a range of fees, often with a minimum cutoff point. Low fees might range from twenty-five to seventy dollars per session. Don't let high fees preclude your seeking treatment. There are many therapists who are sympathetic to economic concerns and the need for affordable treatment.

They can help you locate reasonable options that might be available in your area.

Payment is an important part of therapy. It represents a direct investment in yourself. When therapy is free, it alters motivation. Therapy is seen as more valuable when some effort to pay for treatment is necessary. You may have a tendency to work harder when a financial value is attached to treatment sessions. The tendency to work actively in sessions is reinforced when payment is required. Therapy should require some effort for payment, but the burdens should not be excessive. Therapy should not come at the cost of financial security and economic well-being.

With therapy, it is not necessarily true that you get what you pay for. High fees do not guarantee quality. Some expensive therapists are poor clinicians, and some reasonable therapists are highly skilled. Look to university settings to find a therapist in training. Beginners can be as effective as senior therapists. Certainly, beginning therapists are no worse than experienced therapists. Also, many senior clinicians may take on *pro bono* (courtesy) clients as a way to contribute back to the communities in which they practice. Be wary of therapists who charge excessive fees or require unusual payment arrangements such as payment in advance. Unless some arrangement has been made for third-party reimbursement, fees should be paid at the time of service.

Insurance

Health insurance plans generally include some provisions for treatment of psychological difficulties. Managed-care plans usually require a referral from your primary-care provider, then offer a set number of sessions within that particular plan. Some plans require that you cover a copay amount for services used. Sessions are covered on the basis of medical necessity and demonstrated progress in treatment. Primary-care providers are generally willing to refer a client with psychological distress to a psychotherapy provider. Studies show that when clients receive adequate counseling for emotional needs, they tend to require the services of a medical doctor less frequently.

Traditional fee-for-service plans and preferred provider organizations will generally cover part of the cost of psychotherapy, while you meet a copay for services. Even the best fee-for-service plans generally only cover mental health services at 50 percent. There is usually an annual limit to reimbursement and a lifetime maximum for coverage of services.

Medicare also provides coverage for mental health services. Currently Medicare may pay for services provided by medical professionals other than physicians. In some cases, the services of clinical psychologists or clinical social workers are covered. This coverage may be limited, so call your medicare carrier to find out if medicare will pay for the kind of service you need. Most Medicare subscribers are being shifted to managed-care plans, which provide comprehensive, integrated treatment services. There is generally coverage for mental health care, with an identified provider. Medicare currently also covers psychiatric services performed by a psychiatrist or psychiatric nursing specialist in the home for homebound elderly or disabled clients. In-home services are generally underutilized and should be considered for more homebound clients.

Reimbursement for treatment of emotional disorders has traditionally been paid at a lower rate than for physical disorders. Medical treatment has historically been covered at 80 percent whereas mental health treatment has been covered at only 50 percent.

We might speculate about the reasons for this inequity. Is it possible that as a culture we place less value on mental health when compared to physical health? Do we fail to recognize the connection between mind and body? Do we suspect that people with emotional difficulties are simply malingering? Do we expect clients with emotional symptoms to pull themselves "up by the bootstraps"?

Some advocacy groups in Washington have tried to legislate equal consideration of coverage for mental and physical difficulties. Efforts at national health-care reform have failed to achieve *parity,* or equality in reimbursement patterns. If you are interested in helping to influence legislation for coverage for mental health services, please become active and vocal with local, state, and national policymakers. Write to your representatives. Contact advocacy groups such as the National Alliance for the Mentally Ill (see chap. 14 for address).

Privacy

Privacy is a necessary prerequisite for psychotherapy. You have a right to know that what you say will not be repeated without your knowledge and permission. For the process of psychotherapy to be successful, you must feel confident that what is said will remain private. To feel safe to reveal concerns that may be embarrassing or shameful, a client must have the security of knowing that what is talked about will be confidential. The legal system recognizes this need for privacy and has enacted laws to protect information disclosed during therapy.

Frequency of Visits

In general, you will sense intuitively how often you need to meet with your therapist. Most people begin treatment with ideas about how much support they need or change they wish to accomplish. Even people with little background in therapy have an intuitive sense of how often they need to meet with their therapist. The therapist also will have ideas about how to schedule sessions. The frequency of meetings should be tailored to meet individual needs. For example, initially a client may be in a great deal of distress and wish to meet more frequently. The nature of the work will also influence how often you wish to meet.

It is a good idea to begin treatment with an extended evaluation, scheduling once- or twice-weekly meetings. This can allow you to develop an approach to current difficulties, as well as discuss a schedule for the work. Meeting once a week allows for regular support and provides forty-five or fifty minutes of sustained concentration on the issues at hand. Meeting more frequently allows for added support and more time in-session to concentrate on understanding and changes. Increasing the frequency of meetings can have an exponential effect on the therapeutic work. Meeting more often can allow better recall of material discussed in previous sessions. A continuity develops, and time between sessions increasingly becomes filled with thoughts about the work.

The intensity of the relationship between the therapist and the client increases with more frequent meetings. When sessions are scheduled more frequently, there is ample time to explore both current life situations and recollections of previous events. With increased time in-session, you may be able to talk about experiences in your everyday life and still have sufficient time for introspection or recalling and reworking issues from the past. If the therapy has a behavioral focus, increasing the frequency of meetings may help to strengthen reinforcements and support intensive practice of exercises and new behavior patterns.

The schedule of meetings should be related to the goals of the treatment. If a client is looking primarily for validation and support, meeting once weekly may be adequate. Meeting more frequently allows the client to look at current life events, as well as spend time thinking about where patterns developed, and explore the past. The more frequent the meetings, the more intense the transference, working through, and termination will be.

Some therapies have relatively infrequently scheduled meetings. For example, visits for medication management may occur once every two months and be short in duration (fifteen minutes). Supportive therapy often takes place in weekly meetings. On rare occasions, it may occur monthly or biweekly. Ongoing exploratory psychotherapy requires at least once-a-week meetings, and can meet as often as three times a week. Psychoanalysis, which involves meeting four or five times a week, is an intensive treatment.

Time between sessions is important for working through, reflecting, introspection, and self-exploration. Information uncovered in-session must be incorporated over time. Time between sessions allows for association to current in-session work. Memories may surface, or new perspectives may evolve between sessions. Time between sessions can create opportunities for understanding the effects of separations and an increased awareness of personal boundaries.

What Makes Therapy Successful?

One of the factors that influences the potential for success in therapy is the level of distress that you bring to the treatment. When there is a lot of distress at the beginning of therapy, it may be easier to see rapid changes and improvements. If you are in a great deal of distress when you begin therapy, you may be more motivated to work in the treatment. When feeling better is of paramount importance, you will work to bring issues to sessions and practice new ideas and behaviors between meetings.

Therapy is more likely to be successful if the client believes the treatment will work. If you have a belief that the form of treatment you have chosen is effective, you are more likely to be helped by psychotherapy. This is not merely a placebo effect, which occurs when a person believes herself to have been helped even though the treatment provided was inert.

Rather, when we believe in the possibility of success, we may be more motivated to do the work of change. A belief in treatment efficacy helps to lay a foundation of trust for the collaboration. Trust is a necessary foundation for disclosure, and disclosure is necessary for resolving emotional difficulties. Resolving emotional issues can be arduous work, and if a client believes the treatment will ultimately be successful, they are more likely to dedicate themselves to working toward recovery. Attending sessions and exploring previously warded-off aspects of emotion and personality require an effort. If it is undertaken with a spirit of hopefulness, the energy required to participate flows more easily.

Another factor that influences the success of therapy is the confidence that the therapist has in the process. When a therapist believes strongly in the efficacy of treatment methods, positive effects are more likely to occur. Perhaps the therapist subliminally communicates her hope and optimism to the client. The therapist is increasingly likely to persist through difficult aspects of treatment if she is confident about a positive outcome.

Top Ten Myths About Therapy

1. *"I'm here, now fix me."*
   Therapy does not work on a surgical model. You cannot expect to go to sleep and let the therapist do all the work. The therapist is neither a mechanic, nor a messiah. Therapy requires your active participation in order to see positive effects.
2. *"Why doesn't the therapist just tell me what to do?"*
   If only this were possible. If only the therapist could give

specific instructions and expect them to be followed! Can you imagine saying to someone who is schizophrenic, "Stop hallucinating," or to the person with obsessive compulsive disorder, "Stop checking the stove." Beginning therapists are often tempted to solve problems by telling clients what to do. They quickly learn that clients rarely follow these instructions. I do not give directions because inevitably the client will do something else. The best way to solve a problem is to come up with your own solution. Because you thought of it, and therefore believe in it, you are more likely to follow through with the idea. This may seem a cumbersome process, but it is not possible to *instruct* people out of their symptoms and conflicts. Patterns of behavior are held in place by psychological forces that demand attention. Being told what to do has little impact in the face of these forces.

3. *"The past is the past . . . it doesn't affect me now."*
   It is common for people to discount the impact of previous experiences on current problems. Yet it seems clear that as human beings we are bound by patterns. We are our development. We are our history. Only by acknowledging our previous life experiences can we hope to minimize their impact on the present. Our early experiences and relationships form a prototype for later years. We repeat early experience aspects that are pleasurable, and rework areas of conflict and trauma.

4. *"The therapist is to blame when something goes wrong."*
   At times, it is difficult to evaluate the progress being made in therapy. Anxious or angry feelings may indicate that critical issues are being examined. However, if you find yourself unable to reach the goals of therapy, it may be important to discuss this with your therapist. Client and therapist have mutual responsibility for identifying goals and for making progress toward them.

5. *"Just pick yourself up by the bootstraps."*
   For many people with psychological distress, it is impossible to simply shake off or ignore the distress. Do not confuse ordinary psychological reactions with clinical symptoms. For example, ordinary depression is transient and often related to a specific set of circumstances. Clinical depression persists for weeks or longer and interferes with achieving life's ordinary goals.

6. *"Why can't I just take a pill?"*
   We have been searching for "the magic bullet" since the beginning of time. If only it were possible to create mental health with a pill. Although medications may have a role in improving psychological functioning, they can never be the complete answer. Our minds are not simply biological. In addition, our biology seeks homeostasis. So for most substances we ingest, the body adapts to having these substances on board. Longer-term improvements may be more difficult to achieve if factors other than biology are not addressed.

7. *"Something is morally wrong here."*
   We have a lingering tendency to see symptoms as sins. This is particularly true with addictions. We perceive symptoms as being related to lack of willpower. This attitude limits the possibility for change. The client is condemned rather than helped. If symptoms are viewed as information, then change is possible.

8. *"If I can just uncover the moment that this all started . . ."*
   There generally isn't one trauma or incident—or even one relationship—that started all this. Many people believe that if they could just identify the trauma that is at the root of all the trouble, symptoms would disappear. Symptoms are the result of a process, not an event. Symptoms are multidetermined, meaning they are sustained by multiple causes. They appear in the personality as a result of

layers of experience. Understanding conflicts and symptoms in therapy has been likened to peeling the layers of an onion.

9. *"Talking about things doesn't help."*

While it is true that talking about the past does not change past events, it can change your reaction to these events. Putting thoughts and feelings into words can have a number of positive effects: As you choose words, ideas are clarified and easier to examine. Sharing words with another allows an outside perspective. Shame is decreased. Expressing emotions allows them to be resolved.

10. *"It's all Mother's fault."*

Many people perceive therapy as a witch-hunt, or a search for where to place the blame. While it is true that in therapy we ask, "How did this come to be? What influences contributed to the current situation?" we are looking for understanding, not fault. Parents have a tremendous influence on our personalities. In most families, except where there is constant abuse, this influence is partly positive and partly negative. Most mothers and fathers do a "good-enough" job. However, most families have some dysfunction. When we attempt to understand how your idiosyncrasies might have developed, it is in the hopes that with this awareness, you can take increasing responsibility for your behavior and actions. Once the origins of an issue are identified, the client can forgive parents their shortcomings and take greater responsibility for himself.

Matching Treatment, Client, and Situation

Every individual brings unique conflicts, situations, and characteristics to treatment. There are no easy cookbook rules to follow for matching which type of difficulty will respond best to which form of treatment. Successful therapy depends on effective matching between client, therapist, issue, situation, and developmental levels.

When you begin to work on personal development with a professional counselor, a number of things should be considered: How good is your fit with the therapist? How well does your style match your therapist's style? Are your methods of communicating complementary? Is there an easy rhythm in interchanges? The match between the communication styles of the client and therapist can contribute to a successful working alliance. If there is a congruence in approaches to understanding and an easily shared perspective, exchanging ideas may be more comfortable.

Treatment choice depends on your goals. If you have a well-contained issue that might improve with clarification or simple adjustments, a time-limited, focused therapy might be most appropriate. For example, if you are dealing with grief, you may feel better after several sessions of talking with a counselor. If you need help modifying a behavior, such as improving time management, several sessions may be sufficient.

Most people come to treatment with issues that are more complex and symptoms that are embedded in personality. If your goal is to change life patterns or alter fundamental relationship tendencies, treatment may take somewhat longer. Clients often present a seemingly simple issue, such as being in an abusive relationship, and find out through treatment that this symptom is maintained because of early experiences that contributed to forming character. When the goal of treatment is character change, it make take several years.

Most clients will select therapists who share similar values. Values appear to be more important in a match than physical or demographic characteristics such as age, sex, or race. For example, if a therapist is primarily cognitive and works with modifying thoughts, and a client naturally processes information intellectually, they may work well to-gether by using a cognitive approach. A fundamental belief in the value of thoughts is common to both participants.

Prospective clients frequently ask me about my values concerning spiritual beliefs. It is more common to be asked about my tolerance of spiritual beliefs than about my theoreti-cal rationale for practice. Clients want to know if I understand what it means to be Catholic, or whether I am sympathetic to new age philosophies. A client once asked if I was familiar with Baba Muktananda. Clients sometimes ask if I understand orthodox and comparative religions. Clients and therapists who share common spiritual beliefs may form a good match because they share a common language, as well as common views. However, it is not necessary for a therapist to have any particular spiritual inclination in order for them to understand a client's perspective. The skills required for understanding a client's spiritual beliefs are empathy and listening. A good therapist will learn about the experience of a particular faith or spiritual practice by listening carefully to your description. Understanding can come from sharing the client's feelings and concerns empathically.

Selecting a treatment modality may be more a reflection of the therapist's training than client preference. There is little evidence that one type of therapy is better than another with general symptoms. There is also little support to suggest that length of time the therapist has been in practice is a factor in successful treatment. Some studies show that beginning thera-pists may be more effective because they are likely to ap-proach each client with a great deal of attention and more sensitivity. The benefits of an experienced therapist include having seen many clients, often in a wide variety of circum-stances. There is evidence that therapists who practice using strict adherence to a firmly held theory have better success. For example, a therapist who believes strongly in a cognitive approach and who practices a pure form of cognitive therapy may have better success than an eclectic therapist who borrows techniques from multiple ideologies.

For the most beneficial effect, treatment modalities may need to be combined. For instance, a psychotherapy may be combined with pharmacotherapy to assist with more rapid improvement in symptoms. Cognitive exercises may be combined with sessions devoted to exploring the unconscious.

But Can Therapy Help Me?

You may be wondering if therapy can help with your specific problems. Everyone who comes to therapy is unique. No two issues are exactly alike. Two people may have depression, but that depression may be experienced differently. We bring from our personal history a set of experiences unlike anyone else's. Our personalities are distinct and unique. The techniques of therapy take this individuality into account. However, we can make some general statements about which types of treatment are likely to be most helpful for some specific symptoms.

There are many paths to growth and resolution. I am always wary of someone who purports to have *the way* or *the truth*. There are many different ways to reach the same destination. When you are looking for growth, a path will present itself. You may wish to embrace many methods, or use only a few concentrated techniques. My guiding principle is, "If it works, keep doing it." Therapy can provide one method for resolving conflicts and diminishing the impact of symptoms. Each type of therapy offers some benefits to the client. In general, it has been shown that no one therapy is superior to any other. However, for certain symptoms, some studies have demonstrated that specific types of interventions may be better than others. No matter the method, you may benefit most if you fully participate. You will get out of therapy what you put into it.

Symptoms must be respected. The mind copes with anxiety and adversity using all its available resources. The efforts an individual makes to cope might be simultaneously adaptive and maladaptive even when these efforts result in the expression of symptoms. The mind evolves symptoms from its own perspective as a way to protect itself. At some level, the mind sees symptoms as necessary for survival. The origins of symptoms should be respected and understood before any attempt to remove these symptoms is made. For example, depression may be a defense that the mind uses to quiet its activity. A person may develop depressive symptoms as a way to cope with mental activities that are overwhelming, such as racing thoughts or hallucinations. If the therapist works to remove the depressive symptoms too quickly, the client may become aware of more disturbing symptoms. Given this caveat, we can identify some suggestions for therapy techniques that might be useful with specific symptoms or issues.

Therapy Can Help With . . .

Addiction

If you are wondering about whether you are addicted to a behavior, drugs, or alcohol, it is a good idea to discuss it with a therapist. Addiction might include mood-altering substances, like liquor, wine, beer, street drugs, prescription drugs, over-the-counter drugs, or cigarettes. Addiction might mean a behavior, such as gambling, overeating, shopping, or sex. Addiction is treatable. Recovery is possible. Many forms of support are available to you in your recovery. Long ago, therapists did not like to treat addicts because they did not respond favorably to traditional methods. However, professional care providers have learned how to be helpful to clients in recovery by working conjunction with twelve-step programs, as well as a concentrated scientific effort directed at developing effective treatment interventions for addiction. You may wish to combine a traditional psychotherapy with twelve-step work. Psychotherapy must be tailored to your specific needs dependent on where you are in terms of sobriety. Clients have different needs at different points in recovery. Medications may be a part of treatment for addiction. Family members or adult children of addicts may also benefit from individual or family psychotherapy, or from focused support groups.

Anger

Anger is one of the most troubling emotions of our time. Most clients come into treatment asking for help in dealing with anger. Perhaps it is so troublesome because it is such a common emotion. We feel some level of anger whenever we are deprived or our wishes are thwarted. When we want something and we do not get it, our natural response is to feel frustrated, irritated, or annoyed. We feel guilty when we get angry. We are unsure of how to express anger nondestructively. We may be worried about impulses we see as unacceptable. At times, society or the legal system has given us specific feedback that these impulses are unacceptable.

Talking about angry feelings in therapy may help them become more manageable. Understanding thoughts and experiences that trigger angry feelings can help alter the outcomes of conflicted situations. When anger is accompanied by destructive behaviors, treatment that involves exercises and social-skills training may be helpful. If a person is prone to violence, treatment must be active and immediate. If a person is unable to control violent impulses themselves, then the environment must offer this support, structure, and control.

Anxiety and Fears

Anxiety is one of the most common reasons for seeking treatment. The goods news is that anxiety responds well to treatment. When feelings of anxiety come from underlying conflicts, understanding the nature of these conflicts often makes a resolution readily apparent. A conflict arises when we want opposite things at the same time. For example, we might want to eat something to satisfy a craving, but we also want to abstain from eating because of self-esteem needs for a trim figure. Anxiety can be relieved by making the unconscious conscious and exploring these underlying conflicts. Talking about anxiety can be an effective way to decrease it. Behavioral therapies also show good effectiveness in reducing anxiety. Behavioral techniques generally involve learning relaxation techniques, including self-hypnosis and biofeedback. Some treatments, such as systematic desensitization, involve being exposed to the feared stimulus while in a relaxed state, and gaining mastery over the situation. This can be done by imagining the situation or by being in the actual real-life situation. A number of anti-anxiety medications can be effective, particularly when used on a short-term basis.

Depression

Therapy can effectively alleviate symptoms of depression. Cognitive therapy has been shown to be particularly effective for clients with depression. Using a cognitive approach to identify thoughts that support feelings of depression, and replacing these thoughts with more functional ideas can have a significant impact on symptoms. When depression has its origins in early experiences of loss, or it is caused by anger turned inward, psychodynamic therapy may be most helpful. As you are able to recognize the conflicts that cause depression and talk about the feelings associated with these experiences, feelings of depression are often alleviated. Many medications are available to reduce symptoms of depression. Research shows that a combination of medications and psychotherapy is more effective in treating depression than either of these approaches used alone.

Financial and Career Issues

Psychotherapy can help you clarify your career goals, as well as better understand how you express your identity through your work. Money may be tied to emotion and personality. If you are having chronic difficulties with money, you may benefit from exploring how values about yourself and your financial choices might be influenced by unconscious forces.

Legal Problems

In general, legal problems are best discussed with a lawyer. Your lawyer will know the risks and benefits of discussing your legal issues with a mental health provider. At times, mental health providers will become involved in custody proceedings and can make recommendations about child-rearing arrangements. If there is a criminal complaint, psychologists and psychiatrists often provide recommendations that can influence the course of legal proceedings.

Life-Style Changes

If you are struggling with some behavioral or relationship pattern that is not working, psychotherapy may offer important benefits. Psychotherapy can be a place for examining life-style choices, and the therapist can serve as a support as you make necessary changes. Psychotherapy can help clarify personal values and examine the impact of life-style choices. However, if you are interested in implementing a fitness program, consulting with a personal trainer and a nutritionist may be of greater value. A therapist can help with the psychological issues that impact fitness, but it is not generally a primary focus of therapy.

Memory Changes and Confusion

If you begin to experience memory difficulties, it is important to consult with a mental health provider. The cause of memory difficulties must be determined. Many physical changes can alter memory; these can be managed with medical treatment. If no physical cause is found, it may be that defense mechanisms are creating lapses in memory. Even if a physical cause for memory difficulty is found, some forms of therapy may be useful in helping you to cope with these changes. Family therapy can be useful to members who are helping someone cope with confusion or memory loss.

Ordinary ambivalence about choices or conflicts is different from confusion and can usually be easily sorted out through discussions in therapy. Profound confusion is often accompanied by other cognitive changes, such as memory loss or altered thought patterns. Therapy can offer support and specific techniques for reducing or managing confusion. There are also medications that may slow the progression of confusion, or restore order to thoughts.

Physical Illness

Psychotherapy can be an important part of treatment for physical injury or illness. The illness experience is often a lonely one, and therapy can provide a setting for discussing feelings about the process. Often, when there is a physical illness, a client also feels anxiety, which can be treated in therapy. Having a therapist for support may help you to follow through with recommendations of care givers, particularly when complex rehabilitative activities are required.

Relationship Concerns

Therapy can help with relationship issues in several different ways: If relationship difficulties stem from inner conflicts, individual therapy can help you resolve these issues so you can be free to experience relationships without the influence of remnants of old conflicts. Therapy can impact a relationship directly by taking both parties into treatment and prescribing new ways to relate. Couples therapy can give you a new understanding of what is occurring in a relationship and can encourage new forms of behavior that might improve the ability to relate to each other. If relationship difficulties are due to a skills deficit, it is possible to learn new relationship and communication skills either through individual or group work.

School Difficulties

From kindergarten to college, school presents significant interpersonal challenges. It is an excellent idea to seek consultation for school difficulties. Problems in school might be related to emotions or intellectual abilities. When emotions are interfering with using all your given abilities, dynamic psychotherapy can increase understanding of the difficulty and resolve the conflicts. If a learning disability is interfering with progress in school, specific techniques can be used to support learning style and minimize specific difficulties. When behavior is the problem, interventions to increase the structure of the learning environment can be designed. Rewards and consequences can be used to facilitate better school adjustment.

Self-Esteem

Most people struggle with some feelings of inadequacy and concerns about self-esteem. Many of us just don't seem to feel as good about ourselves as we might. Sometimes we have experienced being powerless or overwhelmed. Psychotherapy can have a profound, positive effect on self-esteem. The experience of having a therapist validate feelings and perceptions often gives you an immediate boost. Understanding the roots of self-esteem difficulties can arise with dynamic psychotherapeutic work. Cognitive behavioral approaches can offer exercises and new ways of thinking that can gradually improve self-image through new experiences.

Sexual Concerns

There are a number of approaches to sexual problems. Any sexual dysfunction should be evaluated by a medical physician in order to rule out a physical cause for the problem. If the causes are psychologically based, inhibitions can be removed through dynamic psychotherapy. Some therapists specialize in sexual problems and use a combination of talking and prescribed activities to be done by the client at home. Sensate focus exercises can help relax you, as well as help you experience pleasurable sensations. Group therapy might be helpful for clients with common issues, such as incest, particularly when the client is struggling with intense feelings of shame. Psychotherapy does not involve direct sexual contact and does not use sexual surrogates.

Spiritual Development

Psychotherapy can be an important aspect of a spiritual path. It can offer a setting for better knowing your inner self. Although psychotherapy can be helpful in spiritual development, it is not usually the primary method for religious and spiritual practices. Psychotherapy can help increase your awareness of your spiritual energy and the good and divine that is within all of us. Spirituality is often an important part of the psychotherapy process. Psychoanalysis in particular, has many qualities in common with the meditation process, as you gain a deeper inner knowing and peace from resolving internal conflicts. Free association can be likened to a meditative process.

Weight Concerns

If you are dissatisfied with your weight, it may be important to examine these concerns with a therapist. If you cope with emotions by eating, a cognitive behavioral approach can help implement more adaptive choices. A dynamic therapy can assist in strengthening coping with emotions. If you are unable to maintain an adequate body weight, or notice destructive patterns, such as bingeing and purging, or you are excessively concerned with restricting caloric intake, it is important to seek treatment immediately.

CHAPTER 2

Healthy Adjustment

What Is Good Mental Health?

Do you know anyone who is "normal"? Is it even possible to be normal? Or desirable? Chances are that if the illusion of normality exists, it is probably because you don't know the person very well. We all have issues. We all have quirks and idiosyncrasies. In fact, it is highly unusual to find a human being who doesn't have one or two official symptoms at play at various times during life. When you get to know someone well enough, their foibles and follies become apparent. In our humanness, we are imperfect.

What might it mean to be normal? Being normal usually means being like others. One way to define normal is with numbers or statistical averages. We call it normal if the characteristic being measured is pretty much like everyone else's. Societal norms or statistical averages may not be the best indicators of optimal adjustment. For examples, in a large city, displays of aggressive driving are becoming commonplace. Although this behavior may be numerically frequent, it is certainly not optimal or desirable behavior. Statistical averages of behaviors might not be the best indicator of optimum mental functioning.

Good mental health must involve not only the absence of symptoms, illness, disease, or injury but achieving the highest levels of adjustment and functioning possible. Good mental health means having the ability to adapt to the demands of everyday life and fully experience the emotions of life. It involves being able to pursue our highest possibilities and actualize our human potential.

Happiness is an essential component of good mental health. The experience of happiness is personally defined. We have our own ideas about what feelings constitute happiness. We are satisfied by different experiences. We judge individually whether we are experiencing enough happiness to suit us. For some people, relationships bring satisfaction; for others it may be realized through accomplishment or material comforts.

However, good mental health does not mean being happy all the time. Ordinary life offers a series of ups and downs, a cycle of positives and negatives. A person may be mentally healthy but still feel sad or anxious. Good mental health involves a balance of experiences, both positive and negative.

Good mental health involves hope for the future and an optimism about our capacity for survival, both individually and globally. A positive outlook about yourself, the world, and the future is an important aspect of mental well-being. Hopefulness and optimism increase our chances of finding solutions to life's problems. We are more likely to keep trying when we believe there is hope.

Good mental health involves flexibility in adapting to life's challenges. This means that we develop an array of coping skills that can be used as circumstance arise. Coping skills are specific mental techniques designed to address the demands of any given situation. For example, problem solving is a coping skill. You might use the problem-solving method to figure out how to respond to work or child-care demands. Coping is a dynamic, evolving process. As new situations in life are encountered, we stretch to develop our range of coping abilities.

Psychiatrist Harry Stack Sullivan suggests that mental health involves awareness of our own interpersonal functioning. He suggests that we might focus on understanding our relationships with others, and using relationships as a medium of study about ourselves. We see ourselves reflected in our relationships. Who we are is, in part, determined by our relationships. When we develop an awareness of these relationship patterns, and of ourselves, Sullivan suggests, we can achieve greater mental well-being.

For Abraham Maslow, a psychologist, mental health involves an ongoing process called self-actualization. In other words, mental health is not a characteristic, it is an approach to life. In his book *The Farther Reaches of Human Nature,* Maslow describes self-actualization as "experiencing fully, vividly, selflessly, with full concentration and total absorption." In this work, he presents his study of optimally functioning individuals in order to better understand our best human capabilities. This was a unique approach at the time, because most of what had been learned about psychological functioning was derived from the study of clients with symptoms and pathological conditions.

Maslow states that "psychologically healthy . . . people are better cognizers and perceivers." In other words, mental health involves thinking and perceiving accurately, realistically, and adaptively. Optimal functioning involves clarity and accuracy of thought, and breadth of perception. This means that we can comprehend our experiences without blocking out positive or negative aspects of reality. Mentally healthy individuals are capable of immersing themselves fully in the opportunities that arise in life. They are able to participate without self-consciousness or inhibition.

Mental well-being is a subjective, highly personalized

experience. In essence, we each judge the satisfaction or deficiency in our own mental health. We appraise our own adjustment. We decide what is an acceptable level of distress or internal conflict. We evaluate our emotional life as satisfying or not. We evaluate relationships and look for ways to improve communication. Those around us may provide feedback, but decisions to make changes in our emotional or psychological functioning generally come from within. Unless our behavior has become dangerous to ourselves or others, it is likely that *we* will be the judge of whether the time has come for intervention. You will decide how much influence you will allow treatment to have, as well as which issues need to be addressed. You are the most important influence in the process of change.

To Love and Work

Traditional psychodynamic definitions of mental health focus on the capacity for love and work. Sigmund Freud suggested that the capacity to love and work is a useful measure of well-being. Some analysts encourage exploring your experiences, strengths, and limitations in the areas of love or relationships, and in work. The capacity for relationships involves an array of interpersonal abilities. Not only is it necessary to be able to relate successfully with others, but it also requires efforts to develop yourself. A sense of self involves your perceptions about who you are and where your influence in the world begins and ends. Love requires having the emotional capacity for attachment and separation, a capacity to experience clearly the self and others. Being able to work involves intellectual, as well as motivational characteristics. Work involves thinking and planning, as well as sustained effort in the face of challenges.

On the surface, this definition may seem too narrow, but there are many potential levels of opportunity in love and work. The capacity for love may involve self-acceptance or commitment to a life partner. The ability to love can expand to involve the community, national, and planet. In its highest form, love is spiritual and involves a higher power. The capacity for work may simply involve meeting basic needs at a subsistence level. Or work may become an opportunity to actualize full creative potential. Through our work, we can express our interpersonal, physical, and cognitive skills.

Self-Acceptance

In her book *Principles of Intensive Psychotherapy,* noted psychoanalyst Frieda Fromm-Reichman suggests that optimal adjustment involves a congruence between self-concept and self-expression. She is referring to developing knowledge of ourselves through introspection and relationships and feeling confident to show our genuine selves to others in the world. When the person we know ourselves to be is the same as the person we show the world, it indicates a comfortable acceptance of impulses, thoughts, and desires. When we are able to accept who we are, we feel comfortable revealing ourselves to others.

Being

Other philosophies focus on *being* rather than doing in evaluating mental health. Taoist and Zen philosophies encourage valuing the here and now of existence over accomplishment. The acceptance of self, or who we are in essence, and a recognition of the importance of individual energy in relation to the larger whole are the result of psychological development. Satisfaction and good mental health are seen as the result of developing awareness and enlightenment. Wisdom and inner peace are seen as the hallmarks of mental well-being.

Noted psychologist Carl Rogers encourages our focus on

existence and being. Rogerian ideas have had a profound influence on the work of many therapists and counselors. Rogers suggests that in an environment of genuine appreciation and respect, human beings will begin to appreciate who they are rather than what they do. If we are exposed to an atmosphere of respect, empathy, and genuine interest in our development, we will evolve to our highest potential. An environment that has some measure of acceptance and unconditional positive regard is necessary for optimal development. Unconditional positive regard is a client's attitude of self-acceptance and an appreciation of who they are. It is seen as a necessary prerequisite for the work of therapy. The therapist gives the client an experience of being valued without condition. Through this experience, the client develops an increased capacity for positive self-regard.

Needs

Maslow identified that human beings are motivated by needs at various levels. Our most basic needs are food, shelter, safety, and security. We have needs for love and belonging. We have a need to see beauty. We have a need ultimately, to use our fullest potential. When our basic needs are sufficiently attended to, we can pursue satisfaction of higher-order needs. Healthy adjustment is dependent on having these needs met to an acceptable measure of satisfaction.

Capacity for Coping

The definition of mental well-being includes an ability to manage the demands and stresses of life's challenges and fully embrace and participate in life's opportunities. Mental health involves being able to utilize intellectual capacities and have access to a wide range of feelings. Mental health involves the capacity to perceive reality accurately and know the difference between right and wrong. This involves resolving legal, social, and moral dilemmas in a complex society. Mental well-being also includes the capacity for relationships that sustain and satisfy individuals, family, community, and ultimately, the planet. These diverse capacities include a wide range of psychological, emotional, and interpersonal abilities. By concentrating on function, it may be easier to determine normal from abnormal mental health. Rather than judging abstract concepts, it is possible to assess the impact of characteristics and conflicts in real-life terms.

Successful adaptation involves developing a wide array of methods of coping that can be used as needed to meet a variety of situations and challenges. Reliance on several coping options alone may limit potential positive responses. As we progress through life, we build a varied set of methods to cope through trial and error in a variety of situations. Having a balanced array of coping options at your disposal increases the chances for successful coping. For example, having the ability to apply emotional, as well as intellectual resources to address a problem will facilitate a solution that addresses a variety of aspects of that problem.

Perceptions

Perceptions of mental health are influenced by culture, age, and personality. Mental health may be viewed as a personal responsibility, an act of fate, or be attributed to the influences of others. Some cultural backgrounds foster a tendency to be stoic and to suppress any complaints about emotional symptoms. Other cultures favor a tendency to express psychological concerns and emotions through somatization or physical changes. Previous interactions with the mental health system shape our opinions about care providers and treatment options. Personality style may determine our ability to undertake health-promoting activities and make positive choices. For example, a person with a strong sense of self-efficacy and personal control is more likely to see well-being as a personal responsibility, making proactive choices. Self-efficacy is a belief that what you do makes a difference. Believing you have control allows you to act in a manner that influences the situation.

Development

Our development, which is comprised of both experience and maturation, has a significant impact on mental well-being. Although there are individual variations as we grow and develop, we progress through a predictable sequence of events that leads from infancy to adulthood, cradle to grave. Physical growth is accompanied by psychological challenges that seem to be designed to move us toward wisdom and contentment. The phases of growth and development have been characterized and analyzed from several important perspectives. A synthesis of ideas that comes from Margaret Mahler, Anna and Sigmund Freud, Harry Stack Sullivan, Erik Erikson, and Jean Piaget is presented here as a background for understanding mental health and well-being.

In each of these phases, the developing child masters new skills and increases the range of emotional and intellectual coping options. Abilities build as the child successfully negotiates developmental challenges. Skills learned in one phase are retained for use in the future. In addition, when a child fails to develop emotional or cognitive abilities either because of trauma or neglect, these compromises will affect the next developmental phase. For example, if a toddler has difficulty with separation anxiety, adapting to the demands of beginning school may be more difficult. Development builds in layers. If the inner foundation has bumps and glitches, outer layers will be less smooth.

Infancy

Earliest life involves a symbiotic relationship between mother and child. Symbiosis means attachment, or existing as one. Attachment is necessary for survival. The care giver and child form a dyad that functions as a single entity. Existence for the infant depends on the availability of a reliable, consistent care giver. The developmental tasks of infancy involve establishing a sense of basic trust about the world. Through experiences with adequate, reliable care givers, the infant develops a core sense that care givers, and thus the environment, will reliably and predictably meet basic needs. The infant experiments with the world and evaluates responses to cries for help. When expression of need is met by consistent care giving, the infant establishes a sense of trust that the world will provide what is needed.

Perhaps because human infants are particularly dependent on others to provide care, they are genetically designed to evoke nurturing responses. Infants have an array of social abilities. They interact through holding and touch. Some theories describe the care giver as having two functions: relating and holding. The face-to-face interactions and mutual communication involve relating. The care giver also offers holding, which involves both physical and psychological containment. When parental holding is secure and effective, the infant feels safe and secure in the world. Infancy sets a prototype for future relationships. Early experiences with care givers serve as a model for what we expect from subsequent relationships. In the first years of life, we form lasting impressions about

ourselves in relation to others and the world. These proto-
types and impressions can have a profound unconscious effect
on our later sense of well-being.

Toddlerhood

The first three years of life involve rapid growth and acquisition of important fundamental psychological capacities. The
infant grows from a state of symbiotic dependence to recognize a separation between self and care givers. The capacity
for empathy has its foundation in these early relationships.
The drama of separation and individuation was studied in
depth by Mahler and her colleagues. Separation individuation
is a lifelong developmental challenge. As we move from being
symbiotically attached to care givers and establish our autonomy, we work on separation. Individuation is the process of
establishing a unique identity in the world.

Initially, as the toddler recognizes separations from the
care giver, anxiety rising to panic may occur. The fears associated with being apart are accompanied by an elation at the
discovery of a unique self. The early discoveries of autonomy
are at once thrilling, stimulating, and frightening. The toddler
experiences a delight in the newly discovered freedom to explore the world. The child explores self-definition through
experimenting with this asserting of his will. This is particularly evident in struggles that arise with toilet issues. The child
asserts personal presence when limits are set, and enjoys frustrating adults with a newly discovered favorite phrase, "No!"
The delight in exploring newfound abilities is interrupted by a
need for refueling and returning to care givers for reassurance
and comfort.

As the child grows into the oedipal years, gender identity
is strengthened, and a set of standards for right and wrong is

internalized. The oedipal years begin during the third year of life and can last until age five or six. By observing children in his family, Freud discovered what he believed to be a universal developmental phenomenon: He noticed that during these years, a male child develops increasing interest in and attachment to his mother. The child attempts to keep the focus of his mother's attention, to the exclusion of others. He comes to see his father as a competitor or rival. The child wishes to destroy this rival so he can have mother all to himself. However, he feels dreadfully inadequate when he compares himself physically with the rival father. Through wrestling with these passionate conflicts and emotions, the child eventually realizes that attempting to destroy his rival might have negative consequences. He begins to feel guilty about these wishes and decides it is better to relinquish the desire for mother in favor of sharing her affections and keeping father present. The child decides that it makes more sense to become like father rather than destroy him. Through this process, the child gains a stronger sense of personal identity and right and wrong. Although Freud believed the attachment to mother was about sexuality, later theorists suggested it was really about possession. It is a desire for having, not for sexual gratification.

For female children, the oedipal drama is somewhat different. The mother is the female child's primary love object. If the girl is to be able to enter into pursuit of affection toward the opposite-sex parent, she must first give up this primary attachment.

Studies suggest that even in same-sex-parent and single-parent homes, children will traverse these developmental conflicts. Children will work through the necessary conflicts with the adults available in the environment. The struggles of the oedipal phase yield a strong sense of identity and a sense of right and wrong. The child learns to renounce destructive or selfish desires for the good of all.

School-Age Child

The age at which children enter organized education programs has been changing. Some children begin in out-of-home educational settings very early, such as in day care. These days, a child rarely stays at home until kindergarten. Whenever the child begins formal or structured group contact with peers and adults outside the family, a new world is discovered.

The world becomes much larger than the immediate family or home unit. School introduces an exciting new element of socialization. As children enter school, peer relationships take on increasing importance, and cooperative relationships are learned. Friendships are formed with same-sex peers, and children begin to explore themselves in relation to the opposite sex.

The school-age child learns about rules that govern the functioning of social groups. As children line up for recess, they are learning about our social contract. Hopefully, the child in school learns that rules facilitate cooperation and ideal outcomes. Feedback from peers and teachers can foster a sense of self-efficacy or ability to tackle life's challenges. The child develops a sense of ability and increasing identity as she interacts with this new world of adults and peers. Ideas that are different from the family's may be encountered.

Adolescence

Becoming a teenager brings rapid physical development, increasing freedom, and confusing sexual changes. During these years, hormones are at a lifetime high of activity. In adolescence, a broader understanding of the world develops, and vocational interests come into focus. Relationships become more sustained and involve the newly interesting element of heightened sexuality. Adolescence may be a challenging time for some, but studies show that for many, these years pass without major disruption. Teens experiment with values and different aspects of identity. They may seem defiant as they challenge existing social rules. These years are often marked by a ceremonial rite of passage into adulthood, either formal or informal.

Adulthood

Traditionally, developmental psychology ended its focus with the attainment of adulthood. However, contemporary perspectives identify phases of development that continue throughout the life span.

Young adulthood involves leaving home and establishing meaningful work and mutually satisfying social relationships. It may involve a marriage or selection of a life partner. Middle adulthood involves the nurturing of children and caring for aging parents. Careers tend to become fully developed and have more meaning and purpose. The mature adult often reaches the peak of his professional contribution and begins planning for the years of retirement.

Aging

Aging has been divided into three distinct phases. The young-old years are often satisfying in terms of having reaped the financial benefits of a career, and rediscovering leisure time through retirement. Health is still generally good, and energy is available for leisure activities. The middle-old person is beginning to slow down. Activities may require more rest and preparation. Health problems may become an issue. The person in the older-old phase often has limited physical abilities. Mental capacities may be retained for some and lost for others to disease processes.

Each developmental phase is important because disruption

in one phase will alter all subsequent phases. If a conflict is left unresolved, a person may become stuck—at least partially—in that phase. The mind struggles for a resolution by repeating the conflict and bringing the issues to the surface. Successfully traversing the variety of developmental tasks and challenges is important in laying the foundation for healthy mental adjustment.

Life's Blueprint

A blueprint is a paradigm we develop for understanding the world. Think of an architect's plans for a building. They may be sketchy, or they can include even the most minute details. The blueprint offers a guide for the placement of each element of the structure, and can later act as a map to find specific areas in the building. The human mind can be viewed as operating with a similar structure and mapping tool. We begin life with a basic genetic ability for developing such a tool. From the beginning, our temperament influences our style. Experiences are logged onto the blueprint much as rooms or additional features might be added to building plans. There are core ideas that make up the center of the structure, as well as areas for unique features. Once the blueprint is in place, most of us move through life collecting evidence that our blueprint is correct and true.

Each person develops life beliefs that are based on personal observations and experiences. Maturation and experience contribute to a personal theory, developed in an attempt to explain everything we encounter. This theory is made up of axioms about life, or conclusions we have made from observation and experience. An example of some of these axioms might be: "life is predictable," or "men are strong," or "women are caring." We form fundamental assumptions about life, such as "I deserve to get what I want," or "I deserve to be loved." These fundamental assumptions gradually form the blueprint for how we conduct our lives. The blueprint is reinforced and validated by information gathered from observations and life experiences.

This blueprint or model that we have of life can be helpful. It simplifies our experience so that we don't need to figure out each situation from scratch. It is a way to organize incoming information, according to experiences we already understand. It allows us the illusion of familiarity. However, the blueprint also limits us. We attend to information that fits into our scheme and ignore contradictory evidence. We cling to our beliefs, convinced of their veracity. To the extent that the blueprint is followed, our experiences are limited. If these guidelines operate below the level of our awareness, we may be destined to repeat the past.

Cognitive psychologists call these blueprints schema, which they describe as patterns of thought or scripts that we follow. The focus is on the concepts of accommodation and assimilation. Accommodation is a cognitive process that involves developing a category for information in our mind. For example, when a child encounters a puppy for the first time, he starts a category of warm, furry beings with wet noses, ears, and tail. When the child encounters a kitten, he is likely to call it a puppy, because it fits most closely with this original category. This is assimilation, or fitting new information into existing mental categories. Since the kitten meows instead of barks, it doesn't quite fit the old category. The child needs to accommodate kittens into a new group. Then as lions, tigers, pumas, lynx, and bobcats are encountered, the process of assimilation and accommodation will build a mental representation of cats that is comprehensive and flexible.

Psychodynamic therapists focus on the forces at play in the personality. Analysts describe our blueprints as unconscious transference and repetition compulsion. They believe that our early relationships are the basis for our relationship paradigms. Repetition compulsion is the tendency to repeat old dramas. The motivations for repetition and transference are complex and usually unconscious. Transference involves reexperiencing old relationships by ascribing aspects of these past experiences onto current, everyday relationships. We may wish to repeat experiences that were initially gratifying in some way in order to have those positive feelings again. Or we may wish to repeat patterns in the hopes of establishing a new outcome or mastering some previously overwhelming challenge. We may play out different aspects of past experiences, taking on roles that previously belonged to others. For example, if a child goes to the doctor, later she may play doctor with her dolls. This is a way to be the one in control of the situation and repair any damage from the indignities of an examination.

We move through life generally unaware that we are influenced by these patterns. When we encounter a new situation, we attempt to find out where it fits in the blueprint. We may mold aspects we observe in order to create an easier fit. Part of the problem with our blueprints is that they may leave us repeating old patterns and missing new opportunities. For example, blueprints have a significant influence on how we experience relationships. Say you encounter an authoritarian, stern, and unfriendly teacher in first grade. The blueprint captures a new plank built on the assumption that teachers are mean and authoritarian. When you enter second grade, the teacher may be lovely, warm, and kind. But because of your blueprint, you mistrust her and look for evidence that she is authoritarian. You relate to her as you did the first teacher because of inherent expectations. This gets tricky, because if you relate in this manner to the second teacher, in response to imposed unconscious expectations, she may actually begin to act more like the first.

Viewing life through the lens of our theory, it is easy to find data that support it as true. What fits our theory is quickly logged and gathered. What doesn't fit is altered to make sense within the theory. For example, if one of your axioms is "Men

are violent," every time we see a man involved in violent behavior, we log it and tally it in our data banks. We may have a
tendency to notice a man's aggressive behavior and highlight it
in our minds. When we meet men who are nonviolent, we may
dismiss this inconsistent data, minimizing its importance or
attributing the behavior to other factors. Not at all scientific,
we move through life looking for data that confirm our belief
that men are violent, and discard contradictory findings, thus
validating an incorrect conclusion.

The Impact of Trauma

An ideal environment for growth and development involves a
reliable care giver who is responsive to the child's needs. Normal development involves inherent, inevitable traumas, and
developmental challenges, such as separation from care
givers. Ordinary life provides experiences that challenge our
capacities for psychological coping. Exceptional events may
present additional demands on existing emotional capabilities.
If the developing child experiences situations that overwhelm
the ego's existing resources for coping, the child will experience subjective distress. As a child moves through the normal
phase of development, vulnerabilities give rise to specific
fears, which correspond to developmental challenges.

As infants, instinctive fears about the absence of a care
giver are most salient. Without a consistent and reliable care
giver, the infant will die. Survival depends on the infant successfully engaging an adult to provide for them. This is accomplished with the aid of certain neurological reflexes, such as
orientation to touch or sound. Even the earliest of social
smiles seems to be a biologically wired mechanism to engage
interaction. The greatest distress in infants occurs when there
is a separation from the care giver. Even the temporary loss of
the care giver results in anxiety. Rene Spitz, a renown child
researcher, studied infants being raised in institutions and

found syndromes of depression and anxiety in infants who had no personal primary care giver. Babies who were not nurtured sufficiently developed failure-to-thrive syndrome. Behavioral psychologist Jean Harlow's studies with monkeys suggest that it is not so much the need for food as the need for nurturing that drives infants to seek comfort in care givers. In his studies, monkeys separated from their mothers were given two substitute care givers, each rigged with a bottle for nourishment. One was made of wire, the other made of cloth. Infant monkeys preferred the soft cloth mother, even when the nourishment was removed. Although we are not monkeys, and ethics do not permit such studies with human infants, child-welfare workers observe similar patterns of behavior in children who are abused: They remain attached to abusive parents rather than face separation.

Trauma need not be so blatant as sexual or physical abuse or neglect. Denial can have a traumatic effect on the growing child. By denial I mean that when a child's natural reactions are shamed or covered up, a part of the child is denied. For example, if a parent says, "That doesn't hurt. Stop crying or I'll give you something to cry about!" the child's pain and natural response to pain are denied. The child is separated from his feelings. Gradually, the message becomes: Deny the pain. As challenges grow more complex, addictive behaviors might be used to help deny whatever pain is present. This person has learned from childhood what I affectionately call the Homer Simpson method of dealing with emotions: "Stuff it way, way down, where it will never be seen again."

John Bradshaw, a contemporary treatment expert in addictions and recovery, calls this soul murder. To some extent, all of us have had parts of our souls murdered. The socialization process requires that some natural reactions be curbed in public. Healing begins when you acknowledge the subtle—and sometimes not so subtle—traumas of having perceptions and emotions denied. We can begin to reconnect with our emotional selves through accepting our own reactions without judgment. In interactions that validate our perceptions, we can begin to reconnect with our inner selves.

Some positive experiences, as well as negative ones may overwhelm coping resources. For example, the thrill of a roller coaster is at once overwhelming and fun. Ticking a child may be enjoyable but can also be overwhelming. More commonly, our emotional resources are overwhelmed by negative experiences. Feelings of fear in response to destructive expressions of anger in care givers may overwhelm a child's capacity for processing emotions and thoughts. When parents lose control of angry impulses and act destructively, a child will feel confused and overwhelmed. Violation of a child's privacy or physical boundaries through physical or sexual abuse will cause the ego to be overwhelmed by confusion and anxiety.

When a trauma occurs, our energy is taken up with coping with the crisis. Work on developmental tasks is temporarily interrupted so that we may deal with the crisis. If events have enough impact, part of our energy may remain caught up in the events, reworking, reliving, and rethinking the trauma. This is called fixation at traumatic points in development. Symptoms later in life may be related to parts of the mind still caught up in these early dramas.

The Development of Thinking

Piaget saw the child as an active participant in the environment, trying to make sense of the world. Eventually, through developing cognitive abilities, the child's coping is facilitated and she gains mastery over the environment. Piaget suggests that as the child encounters a new situation, she tries to understand how it all works. Through observation and mental manipulation, the child evolves rules about how the world operates. At various stages of development, thinking is governed by these rules. The child builds cognitive abilities as she begins to understand the logic of the world through concepts such as time, speed, space, logic, number, geometry, and movement. Piaget identified changes in our thinking that occur in predictable phases throughout development. He called these phases sensorimotor, preoperational, concrete operations, and the stage of formal operations.

The sensorimotor phase encompasses birth to two years. Language and the symbolic use of sound appear. The child experiments on the world through moving it, and by observing consequences. He learns through feeling, smelling, tasting, and hearing. Object permanence is a kind of memory system. During this phase, the child develops an ability called object permanence, or the ability to hold a mental representation of a person or object in his mind, in the absence of that person or object. Object constancy develops as the child is able to see that people contain both good and bad properties. Images of people as all good or all bad are relinquished as the child realizes that sometimes people are good, and sometimes they are bad.

The preoperational phase lasts from approximately ages two to seven and is characterized by the development of the use of symbolism and fantasy. Children in this phase are unable to understand reciprocity. For example, a child may say that although she has a sister, she may not recognize that her sister also has a sister. There is difficulty seeing the world from another's perspective.

During the age of concrete operations, a child learns several rules about the operation of the world. These include conservation and reversibility. For example, a child who is preoperational may see two ounces of water in a short, fat cup as having less volume than two ounces of water in a tall, skinny cup because the water level in the tall cup is higher. Once a child reaches concrete operations, he can pour the two ounces of water into differently shaped cups and realize that the volume of water remains the same. Concrete operations need to be here and now, and observable.

During the formal operations stage, the child develops the ability to manipulate mental representations without having them present in physical reality; he can also work on abstract concepts. During adolescence, the child develops an increasing ability to think about abstract concepts and work symbolically. Advanced analytic skills continue to develop with new intellectual challenges.

Personality and Emotions

Personality is the expression of who we are. But what is it and what constitutes who we are? Scientists and philosophers have studied personality from many different perspectives. The study of personality is often fragmented and has been heavily influenced by personal interests. It has been likened to several blind men studying an elephant with their hands. One man feels the ears and describes a fan. Another feels the tail and says it is a brush. Another feels the leg and describes a tree. Each person who studies personality does so through the lens of their own. Explanations about who we are are colored and shaped by who we are.

Most of us have a personal theory about what makes up personality. What is your definition of personality? Which do you believe has more influence: biology or experience? Do you think that developmental history influences personality more than current circumstances? Do parents play a role in who we eventually become? Is parental influence explained by genetics or learning and observation? How much does a situation alter our behavior?

The scientific and philosophical traditions have attempted to explain personality. Some clinicians have focused on attempting to describe and categorize personality traits.

Others have studied personality development and functioning. Much of what we understand about personality comes from work with symptomatic and disordered personalities.

Personality styles show wide variations, as do emotional responses. Our emotions provide significant opportunities and challenges. If we have learned to accept our feelings by having our perceptions validated by significant others, we will be more accepting of our emotions as adults. When feelings are talked about freely, a child learns to identify different emotional states and how to cope with emotional changes. Being able to recognize our feelings is a cognitive skill that can be developed through therapy. Relationships offer experiences with emotions and provide opportunities for learning about ourselves through intimacy with others. Once feelings are identified and labeled, coping with a variety of emotional states can increase with awareness. Talking about feelings may discharge them, as can expression in the arts. Physical activity might present options for coping with emotions. The use of mood-altering substances can become a part of a maladaptive coping pattern because of the immediate results encountered with ingestion of these substances. We can learn what comforts and quiets our emotions, and implements calming techniques when necessary. We learn that if we are observing our emotions, we will never be wholly consumed by the play of these forces. We can observe our dramas with a sense of humor.

Some people will acknowledge physical symptoms long before admitting to any psychological distress. There may be a tendency to express stress or anxiety through physical symptoms. For example, a child may complain of an upset tummy rather than say he is afraid to go to school. If you were raised in an environment where feelings were validated and responded to in a satisfying way, you may be better able to describe and respond to emotional states as an adult.

Most people who enter a therapist's office are struggling

with emotions and emotional conflicts. Intense emotions are often difficult to bear. Even positive emotions can be overwhelming. Anger is particularly troublesome. Many people were exposed to destructive expressions of anger in childhood, and cultural taboos against expression of anger leave lingering feelings of guilt whenever anger interrupts our awareness. Grief over loss is also a difficult feeling to experience fully. Fear is a troublesome emotion. Even intense feelings of love can overwhelm cognitive resources. When we experience conflicting emotions, anxiety may be the result. Defenses against anxiety serve to protect us from these unpleasant experiences.

Behavior

In addition to thoughts and feelings, our personality is reflected in our behavior. Our actions are an expression of who we are. Behaviorists believe that our actions determine our thoughts and feelings, and what we learn from our experiences is the most important factor in forming our personality. These beliefs stem from the idea of *tabula rasa,* which says that all people are born as a blank slate and that personality and behavior are learned through experiences that reinforce certain personality attributes.

Learning theory suggests that we arrive in the world created equally. And given an optimal environment, we can grow to be self-actualized, productive, happy adults. Experiences that cause pain may give rise to antisocial or destructive behaviors. B. F. Skinner suggested he could make a criminal or a success out of any baby simply by altering the environment in which they grew up and by providing different learning experiences. Behaviorists minimize the importance of genetic and biological differences. They see personality as a result of environmental reinforcers that shape behavior.

The main tenets for behaviorism suggest that behaviors that are rewarded are likely to be repeated. Actions that bring negative consequences will diminish. The mind can be understood in the context of a system of reward-and-punishment stimuli. Behaviorists examine the relationship between stimulus, organism, and response. The stimulus is whatever is found in the environment. The organism refers to the person and/or subject and its unique psychological and physical functioning. The response is whatever behavior results from the interaction of the stimulus and the organism.

Biology

The brain makes mind possible. Mind cannot exist without brain. There is no doubt that the physiological structure of the brain has a huge impact on how mind is expressed. Much of what we understand about the importance of the biology of the brain comes from research with clients who have alterations in brain structure and functioning. One of the first clients to be studied was Phineas Gage, an easygoing, hardworking, sociable man. While he was working as part of a railroad-building crew, an accident caused a rail spike to shoot through his chin, up into the middle of his skull. This caused a small tunnel injury that severed many connections between his brain's frontal and parietal lobes. Gage recuperated quickly, but the accident had a profound effect on his personality. After the accident, he was ill-tempered and impulsive. He was given to excessive displays of emotion. Gage inadvertently made a significant contribution to our understanding of the importance of the structure of the brain in personality.

Some of the difficulty in understanding brain mechanisms stems from the limitations of our methods of science. Historically, we studied brains of organisms that were dead. From the time of Leonardo da Vinci, anatomical drawings relied on the study of cadavers. Cadavers are good for learning about the existence of structures. The brain has been well mapped in terms of physical characteristics. However, understanding what these structures do, and how they affect our experience has only recently become a focus. Newer imaging techniques such as positron emissions scanning (PET) and radioisotope tagging have allowed us to see the brain in action, and to speculate about how it works.

In addition to studying people with normal functioning, we have also learned a great deal from studying clients with abnormal brain structures. That is to say, we can observe changes in behavior, then obtain measurements and images of indicators of brain functioning, and speculate about behaviors controlled by that region of the brain. Difficulties with this line of inquiry are that most behaviors require several areas of the brain to function together. Interruption or damage in any one of these areas can interrupt behavior patterns.

The brain is made up of several layers of specialized nervous tissue. The brain is divided into hemispheres or sides. The two halves of the brain are connected by a bundle of nerves called the corpus callosum. The left and right side of the brain seem to be involved in some different behavior and thought patterns. Starting at the top of the nerves that comprise the spinal cord, the brain stem supports involuntary behaviors which are necessary to sustain life: breathing, regulation of homeostasis, and transfer of impulses to higher brain regions. Farther up the nerve tract is the cerebellum, which is involved in balance and coordination of movement. Moving up from the brain stem is an inner brain region that consists of subcortical areas, including the limbic system, amygdala, thalamus, hypothalamus, and pineal gland. (See Figure 2-1.) Many of these structures produce hormones or neurotransmitters that can affect behaviors and emotions. These structures control emotion and drives such as hunger, anger, satiety, elation, or pleasure. This area of the brain regulates primitive survival aspects of behavior. The inner brain is covered by an outer layer called the cortex. Each half of the brain cortex is divided into four lobes: frontal, temporal, parietal,

Figure 2-1 | **Structure and Function of the Brain**

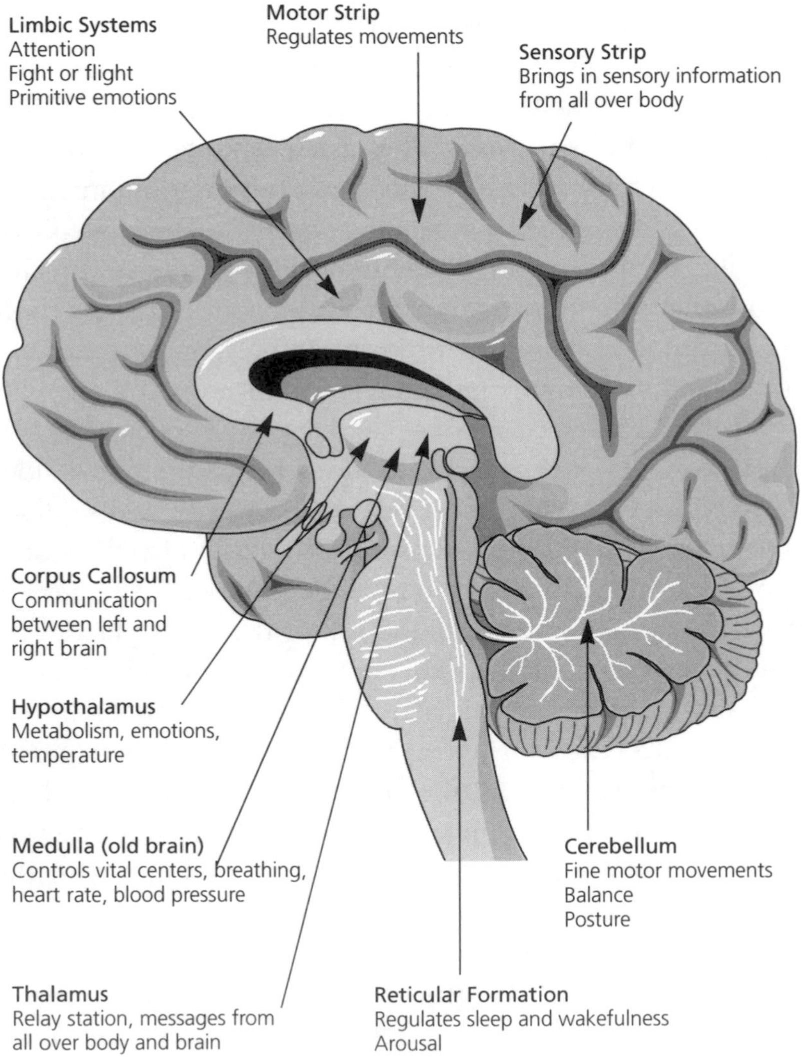

Limbic Systems
Attention
Fight or flight
Primitive emotions

Motor Strip
Regulates movements

Sensory Strip
Brings in sensory information
from all over body

Corpus Callosum
Communication
between left and
right brain

Hypothalamus
Metabolism, emotions,
temperature

Medulla (old brain)
Controls vital centers, breathing,
heart rate, blood pressure

Cerebellum
Fine motor movements
Balance
Posture

Thalamus
Relay station, messages from
all over body and brain

Reticular Formation
Regulates sleep and wakefulness
Arousal

and occipital. Something is known about biophysiological functioning of each of these regions, but there is still much to explore.

The frontal lobe consists of areas that influence higher aspects of a human being. This lobe is involved in planning, abstract thinking, calculations, and reasoning. The frontal lobe inhibits responses that might be inappropriate or antisocial. The frontal lobe is involved in inhibition of expressions of aggression and sexuality, and control of impulses.

The temporal lobe, located adjacent to the ears, is involved in processing auditory information and memory. It also plays a smaller role in processing emotions transmitted from the inner brain regions.

The parietal lobe is involved in the integration of information from the senses of the nervous system. It is also involved in a person's ability to navigate spatial relationships, including movement and graphic abilities.

The occipital lobe is primarily involved in vision. (See Figure 2-2.)

Brain tissue has an amazing quality that is unlike other organ in the human body. It has a quality called plasticity, which suggests that when some forms of damage occur, areas adjacent to or remote from the damaged area may take over functions once influenced by the damaged regions. To a certain extent, if limited damage occurs, the brain can use alternative areas to influence behavior and thinking. This is important because efforts at rehabilitation after injury should include stimulation of cognitive and emotional abilities.

In addition to the brain's physical structure, there are chemicals in the brain and the body that have a profound impact on mental and emotional functioning. These chemicals include neurotransmitters such as norepinephrine, serotonin, and dopamine, and hormones such as cortisol, thyroxine, and adrenaline. Chemical activities affect feelings of well-being, anxiety, and mood.

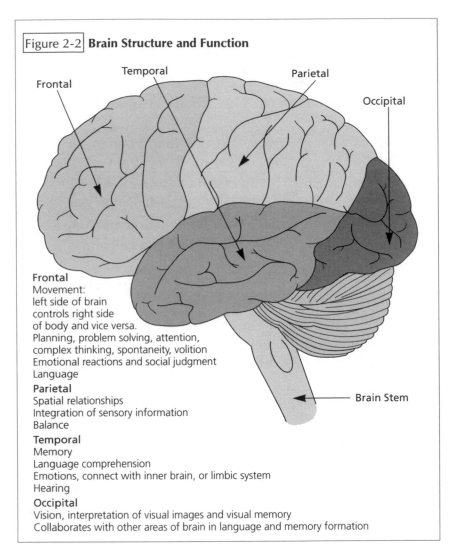

Figure 2-2 | **Brain Structure and Function**

Frontal

Temporal

Parietal

Occipital

Frontal
Movement:
left side of brain
controls right side
of body and vice versa.
Planning, problem solving, attention,
complex thinking, spontaneity, volition
Emotional reactions and social judgment
Language

Parietal
Spatial relationships
Integration of sensory information
Balance

Temporal
Memory
Language comprehension
Emotions, connect with inner brain, or limbic system
Hearing

Occipital
Vision, interpretation of visual images and visual memory
Collaborates with other areas of brain in language and memory formation

Brain Stem

The brain is also alive with electrical activity. Some have suggested that thoughts are actually energy that travels along a neuronal pathway, causing changes in brain structure as they travel. Each time there is a thought, a new neuronal pathway is laid down. If the thought is repeated, the pathway is retraced and thus strengthened.

It is not clear which comes first, the structure of the brain or the function of the mind. The mind and brain seek homeostasis and exhibit many compensatory self-regulating mechanisms. For example, if dopamine receptors are less active, the body may produce larger amounts of dopamine to achieve the same effects.

Dynamic Forces in the Mind

To better understand mental health, it may be useful to explore the structure of the mind and personality. Freud offered a model to understand the dynamic structure and function of the mind. He suggested that we are born with the capacity to reflexively meet survival needs with a mental structure he called the id. It consists of forces that attempt to satisfy basic drives: hunger, need for contact, and expression of dissatisfaction. This part of the mind is governed by the pleasure principle and has an "I want it and I want it now!" kind of attitude. This part of the mind forms a basic core designed for survival and is carried with us all of our days. The id is tempered by the development of the ego.

Through the process of maturation and experience, the ego develops our psychological capacities for thinking and feeling. The ego is the part of the mind that uses logic to organize information about the world, as well as solve problems. The functions of the ego include language, vision, memory, hearing and movement, the ability to play, plan, and manage emotions with thoughts and ideas. The ego manifests defenses that protect us from being overwhelmed by anxiety. The ego manages both internal psychological forces and the demands of the environment. It helps us cope with inner conflicts and the demands of external reality.

During our middle childhood years, Freud suggested that we experience universal human conflicts that encourage the development of a conscience. Through the drama of the oedipal phase (see development section) we relinquish selfish needs in favor of lasting relationships that sustain our sense of security. This process gives rise to the superego and standards of right and wrong. Self-concept is internalized. The superego is the part of the mind that provides conscience and a sense of humor. Freud's structural model is just one way to conceptualize mental functioning, and can be useful for discussing dynamic forces at play in the mind. (See Figure 2-3.)

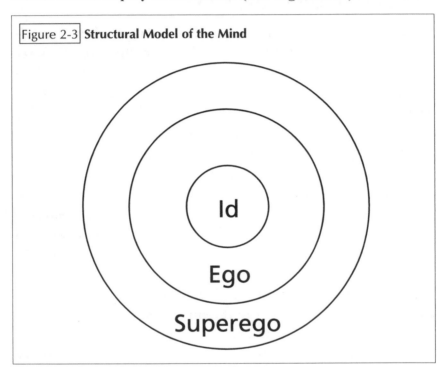

Figure 2-3 **Structural Model of the Mind**

Id

Ego

Superego

Levels of Awareness

In addition to the structural model of the mind, Freud offered a topographical model of thinking that involved levels of awareness. (See Figure 2-4.) He suggested that there are three areas of mental activity: conscious, preconscious, and unconscious. Conscious thoughts are those things that we are aware of in our alert, awake experience. When we say thinking or thoughts we are generally referring to things in our active awareness. Preconscious mental activity is not immediately in

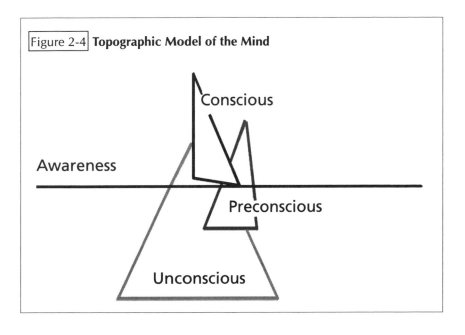

Figure 2-4 | **Topographic Model of the Mind**

Conscious

Awareness

Preconscious

Unconscious

awareness but can be easily brought to mind. For example, if you are asked to describe the temperature of your surroundings or the light in your current setting, although you may not previously have been focused on these environmental characteristics, they can easily be brought into focus. Likewise, if you are asked about your mother's maiden name or events from your childhood, they can be brought into awareness with little effort. According to Freud, unconscious mental activities make up the majority of our psychic processes. Unconscious processes occur outside the level of our awareness. We can only become aware of unconscious processes with a great deal of effort. We must look for clues to the existence of unconscious forces, such as slips of the tongue or dreams. Unconscious activities are difficult to observe directly, but it is possible to relax our awareness in order to allow for greater expression of these ideas. This is done through free association, where the critic is quieted and you say whatever comes to mind. By studying this stream of consciousness, we might often pick up elements of unconscious forces by evaluating patterns. These activities, which exist beyond our awareness, have a profound influence on behavior, thinking, and feeling.

Ego Functions

Recall that the ego is the part of the mind that manages internal forces and the demands of the environment. It balances the variety of psychological forces that come from id wishes and superego admonishments. In addition, the ego helps us negotiate the real demands of everyday life. The functions or abilities of this part of the mind have been studied by psychiatrists and psychologists. Twelve distinct ego functions have been identified and will be discussed briefly because these abilities contribute to good mental health.

The ego helps you perceive reality accurately. It allows you to differentiate which stimuli are coming from the environment (or without), and which arise from your own thoughts (or within). When this ego function is impaired, a person might see or hear things that other people do not see or hear (hallucinations). The ego develops the capacity for judgment and is able to reason through, to see the ultimate consequences of an action. The ego helps manage feelings, wishes, and the expression of impulses. For example, it is an ego function to be able to identify emotions and label what you are feeling. To recognize "I am sad" or "I am scared" is a function of the ego's abilities. The ego allows us to have relationships, partly because it helps us develop an accurate sense of self. It also involves the mental ability to form a cognitive picture of the person in our mind, even though the person is not present. This is called a mental representation. When we are alone, we often do not feel alone because in our mind we remember the people who are important to us. The ego governs our thought processes. It provides logic and order to our thinking. When this function is impaired, such as in schizophrenia, a person's thoughts may become incoherent.

The ego is flexible and can suspend its impact on the mind temporarily so that we might enjoy the benefits of play and creative thought. The ego can temporarily suspend the rules of logic and reason in order to facilitate relaxation. This is called the ability to regress in service of the ego. We are able to let go of some of the demands of logical adult life and laugh or daydream again like a child. This ability also involves being able to return to mature forms of thinking as desired.

The ego maintains a protective barrier to limit the amount of stimulus perceived by an individual. The ego sets the level at which a stimulus will be noted, and a level at which the stimulus will be filtered out. The ego also provides many of the functions that allow us to negotiate our world. These include perception, memory, language, intentionality, hearing, productivity, concentration, vision, motor development, attention, speech, and expression. The ego allows us to integrate complex information and synthesize new ideas. It also facilitates a sense of competence and mastery through experience.

Healthy ego functioning is a necessary prerequisite for optimal mental health. When the ego develops its capacity for these functions, id impulses are controlled and the superego's commentary is quieted. You are then more easily able to address the challenges of daily life and have a wide array of abilities available to use toward self-actualization.

Conflict

Conflict is wanting two different things at the same time. Because the various parts of the mind (id, ego, and superego) have somewhat different aims, they are often at conflict with each other. For example, if the ego gives in to the id's demands for gratification, the superego may react by invoking feelings of guilt. If the ego follows superego mandates, the id may be left wanting for satisfaction and expression of basic drives. In addition, when they are not congruent with our personal desires, the demands of reality might introduce further conflicts. To cope with the anxiety produced by this constant conflict, the ego utilizes defense mechanisms.

Defenses

Defenses are an important aspect of the ego's functioning. I once had a client say, "I don't want to have any defenses!" Defenses are, in part, a good thing. Defenses protect us from anxiety. Without defenses we would be overwhelmed by anxiety and fears. Defenses develop, along with the ego, through maturation and experience. When we are born, our defenses are essentially just reflexes. In our early years, our defenses are primitive and include denial, repression, and projection. As we move through toddlerhood, our repertoire of defenses expands to include splitting and reaction formation. As we move through the oedipal years, we learn projective identification, sublimation, and suppression.

Defenses are both adaptive and maladaptive. For example, repressing an image that is disturbing and produces anxiety is helpful because you are no longer aware of being disturbed by anxiety. However, forgetting the disturbing event may tie up psychic energy—the energy needed to keep this memory out of consciousness makes energy unavailable for other mental activities. Also, being aware of the disturbing event may allow for some correction to take place.

Here is a brief description of some mechanisms of defense, as well as examples of them in action.

Denial is a commonly observed defense. It involves negating some reality. It is evident in the toddler who spills a glass of milk then says, "I didn't do it!" Another example of denial is commonly seen in clients who are addicted. When the addict is unable to see that regular, destructive use of substances is a problem, this is denial.

Projection is another intrapsychic mechanism for quieting our anxiety. It involves attributing some unwanted aspect of our own personality to others and denying it in ourselves. For example, if you are angry and unconsciously believe that anger is an unacceptable emotion, you may unconsciously, automatically ascribe this anger to others rather than acknowledging it in yourself. You may see others as frequently being angry with you and deny that you have any of these feelings yourself. Projection is also involved when we superimpose our mental images of previous relationships onto people we encounter in the present. For example, of our past mental image of teachers is authoritarian, we may see current instructors as being authoritarian, while in reality the teacher may be quite egalitarian. If our experiences with police officers have been negative, we may see any encounter with the police as negative, even if it is polite and uneventful.

Reaction formation is a fascinating mental mechanism. It involves reframing feelings that are unacceptable by making them the opposite of how you really feel. For example, you might unconsciously deny any negative feelings and concentrate only on the positives. For example, if you encounter someone whom you dislike and fawn and gush greetings of warmth, this is reaction formation.

Rationalization involves developing an intellectual explanation for behaviors or feelings. For example, you might explain that you couldn't study for a test because there was so much laundry to do. This reason for not studying ignores any underlying test anxiety that might have been present.

Repression is a universal defense mechanism. It is the automatic barring from consciousness any psychic event that is overwhelmingly traumatizing. The mind automatically eliminates psychic events that are overwhelming. They are hidden in the farthest reaches of our unconscious and can be recalled only with the greatest effort. For example, the mind usually protects us from awareness of destructive or lustful wishes that would arouse anxiety and guilt if allowed into consciousness.

Suppression is similar to repression, but it is a conscious process. Suppression is deciding consciously not to think about some issue or event. For example, concentrating on the present rather than a past traumatic event may involve suppression. As a way to resolve grief, you might decide to think about today rather than dwell on the loss.

Displacement involves transferring feelings about one situation or person onto another situation or person. For example, if you feel angry at your boss but expressing these feelings might jeopardize your employment, you might come home and yell at your dog. The focus of the emotions changes, but the expression of the emotion remains the same.

Sublimation is a mature defense mechanism. It involves taking primitive urges for gratification or expression of aggression and channeling them into socially acceptable behaviors. For example, someone who gets sexual gratification through exhibitionism might become a performer in order to achieve satisfaction for these impulses. This is a socially sanctioned and generally rewarded behavior. If the person were to expose themselves in public, the gratification of these wishes would bring serious negative consequences. Aggressive impulses can also be sublimated effectively. Our vocational choices sometimes offer an example of sublimation. For example, someone who is gratified by displaying physical power over others might become a police officer or a boxer rather than becoming an assaultive criminal. Someone with aggressive urges might join the military.

Defenses operate automatically and often unconsciously. When defenses fail, we see the emergence of anxiety symptoms such as neuroses or psychoses. When we increase our awareness of ourselves and become skilled at looking for indicators of defensive functioning, we can modify our responses to various situation. The goal is not to have no defenses. The goal is to have effective defenses. The goal is also to have a wide variety of defensive strategies from which to choose in any given situation. Pathology results when someone relies too heavily on one or two mechanisms, particularly when these are primitive defenses.

Each of these perspectives contributes an understanding of what helps us develop and maintain good mental health. The structure and function of the mind determine how well we can cope with life's challenges. Our development, personality, thinking, and emotions shape who we are. Our biology and behavior are inextricably linked to influence our mental health.

Now let us look at what happens when there is psychological distress.

CHAPTER 3

Psychological Distress

We are "much more simply human than otherwise."

— Harry Stack Sullivan, *Conceptions of Modern Psychiatry*, 1940

In psychology, we frequently find ourselves thinking about abnormal behavior or maladaptive symptoms rather than good mental health. It is easier to identify behaviors and characteristics that are abnormal rather than define what is normal. When a behavior is unusual or different from the mainstream, we may say it is abnormal. We consider a behavior abnormal if it is maladaptive or produces ineffective results. When behavior is self-defeating or ineffective, it may be labeled abnormal. If behavior becomes dangerous to oneself or others, we call this abnormal.

Concerns That Prompt Treatment

Why do people thing about starting therapy? It has become increasingly acceptable to seek treatment for psychological and emotional difficulties. The types of concerns that may prompt a person to seek treatment include relationship difficulties, work anxiety, management of anger, stress, or fear. Issues related to addiction frequently prompt counseling. When children have conflicts with parents, treatment may be initiated. When medical concerns arise, a counselor may be helpful in managing emotional states associated with the diagnosis and treatment.

Asking for Help

Whether someone chooses to seek professional intervention is influenced by a number of factors. A primary factor that motivates treatment is the client's subjective level of distress. When we are in great distress, we are willing to consider assistance from sources we would not normally utilize. If the pain is significant, we are willing to try almost anything to alleviate these feelings. A second factor involves perceptions about usefulness of treatment. Availability of treatment and cost are factors. Stigma associated with mental health difficulties is a concern that may inhibit seeking treatment. At times, it is not so much the client as the people around the client who are in distress and negatively affected by the client's behaviors. For example, someone addicted to alcohol may have little subjective distress as long as alcohol is readily available. The family may be left to deal with the negative consequences of chronic intoxication in their loved one. In these cases, it is often the family that initiates investigating treatment options.

Asking for help presents interpersonal challenges in itself. The ease with which we can reach out to others in times of confusion and need relates to a basic sense of trust. If we have developed a belief that others will support us as needed, we will feel more confident about reaching out for help. The decision to seek professional counseling adds a dimension to our support system that was not so widely available in previous eras. Since the Victorian era, talking therapies have been available, but they have been primarily utilized by wealthier socioeconomic groups.

The Meaning of Symptoms

The appearance of symptoms has important meaning. Symptoms need to be understood in the context of all mental activity. According to Freud, symptoms "have a connection with the life of those who produce them." The mind constructs symptoms as a way to cope with anxiety and promoting survival. Understanding the causes of a symptom can help you to know how to approach the difficulty.

Symptoms deserve respect and merit considerable study before attempts to remove symptoms begin. Naturally, there are exceptions for symptoms that may be life threatening, but for the most part, it is best to examine symptoms carefully before interventions begin. For example, depression is a common complaint in psychotherapy. The therapist and client must examine the depression to understand its purpose and function within the personality. For some people, depression may be adaptive if it is used to organize the mind. Depression, with its relative monotone, might be preferable to other emotions. If the client has intense emotions that might be chaotic or potentially overwhelming, the dullness of depression may be, in part, welcome. The client may feel overwhelmed if the therapist attempts to remove the depressive symptoms too quickly. Sufficient supports need to be in place to protect the client as symptoms are removed. As coping improves, the symptom of depression used as a defense may become obsolete and fall away naturally.

Compromise Formation

Symptoms are the result of something known to dynamic therapists as compromise formation. When a client experiences unconscious conflicts in emotions and thinking, anxiety and distress can be the result. A compromise formation may allow for different parts of the conflict to be resolved or satisfied at the same time. The compromise allows the various forces to satisfy some of their opposing aims simultaneously. For example, someone who is anxious about intimacy might restrict relationships to people who are unable to form intimate relationships. Although these relationships never fully satisfy longings for true intimacy, the wish for closeness is partially satisfied. At the same time, the anxiety about closeness is quieted because true intimacy is avoided. The symptom that results is dissatisfaction about interpersonal relationships. But an equilibrium has been established to keep the various desires in the conflict at least partially satisfied.

Learned Responses

Symptoms may also be a learned response. We learn through experience and the reactions of others which behaviors elicit positive and negative reactions. We are taught by interacting with significant others how to express emotions and work through conflicts. We learn first from our families, then from our communities which emotions are acceptable, as well as how to communicate them appropriately. We see our parents cope with everyday living and thus learn what options are available. Our teachers have limitations and challenges of their own. If their own emotional and psychological functioning has been impaired, their ability to pass on effective coping patterns may be inadequate. For example, if parents are prone to destructive displays of anger, children will learn that destructive anger is acceptable—and frightening. They may be prone to inhibition of their own anger or to destructive displays of their own.

Physical Changes

Symptoms may also be the result of some change in physiological or biological functioning. We have been able to identify symptoms that correspond to altered levels of brain chemicals, altered brain electrical activity, and altered brain structure. Hormones, metabolic imbalance, and physical illness can produce psychological and emotional symptoms. Genetics plays a role in some individuals' vulnerability to developing psychiatric symptoms.

When a physical component to psychological symptoms is suspected, it is important to incorporate these aspects into plans for treatment. Restoring biological functioning can alleviate symptoms directly. However, when working within physiology, you must keep in mind the body's tendency toward homeostasis. Whenever you alter physical functioning, there will likely be a reaction to the intervention. Side effects must be considered carefully, and provisions made to support long-term progress. For example, although the neurotransmitter dopamine has been linked to experiences of hallucinations, treatment with antipsychotic drugs must be used in conjunction with environmental support that reduces situational anxiety. The body may adapt to medications through homeostasis and render them less effective over time.

Symptoms Requiring Clinical Attention

You may wish to see a counselor if you are currently experiencing any of the following:

_____ depressed mood or feeling blue for more than two weeks.

_____ thoughts of suicide or self-harm

_____ violent impulses or destructive expressions of anger

_____ worries that last more than two weeks or that are unrealistic

_____ frequent arguments with significant others

_____ difficulty maintaining employment or progressing in school

persistent concerns about weight or eating patterns

_____ fears about physical health despite the absence of physical symptoms

_____ ongoing substance use despite the knowledge that it is self-damaging

_____ difficulty concentrating or lapses in memory

_____ shame or confusion about sexual impulses

_____ seeing, smelling, or hearing things that other people do not see, smell, or hear

_____ relationships that are consistently disappointing

_____ unwanted repetitive thoughts or visions

_____ family difficulties

_____ persistent feelings of anxiety

When Seeing a Therapist Is Not Appropriate

When your own efforts to resolve the situation are working, it is not necessary to see a therapist. When difficulties are transient and don't interfere with life, therapy is not necessary. If a problem is likely to be time-limited, or is situation-specific, a long-term therapy may not be needed. When problems relate to maturational crises, generally speaking, they will resolve without professional help.

Diagnostic Categories

Our health system places tremendous importance on diagnosis. Indeed, knowing a diagnosis is helpful in several ways: A specific diagnosis allows clinicians to communicate with each other about etiology and treatment. When diagnostic categories are clearly defined, research design is more accurate, and statistics between groups can be reliably compared. Third-party payment is dependent on having a diagnosis.

However, there may be drawbacks to establishing a diagnosis, or in labeling a behavior as abnormal. In general, we seem to fear clients who have emotional difficulties. Clients who are given a diagnosis may be stigmatized. They may be seen as threatening or defective. When we diagnose a behavior, we officially label it as a problem and treat it as an illness, which ought to be cured or alleviated. When diagnosis involves emotional or mental processes, inevitably subjectivity comes into play.

The history of how to categorize homosexuality illustrates the value judgments that may be involved in making a psychological diagnosis. Psychology and psychiatry struggled for years over how to categorize homosexual behavior. During the 1950s, homosexuality was logged in beside a long list of sexual deviations. Clinicians who saw homosexual clients were encouraged to attempt to alleviate this symptom and promote heterosexual adjustment. We have since recognized homosexuality as a normal variation in adjustment rather than a psychological disorder. New on the horizon, Premenstrual Syndrome recently made it to the list of psychiatric disorders despite protests from women's groups that hormonal fluctuations are normal biological processes.

Although it is illegal, there may be ramifications to having a mental health diagnosis in employment settings. Mental illness is poorly understood by many and may have an impact on perceptions of coworkers and bosses. There may be an impact in insurance coverage for clients who have received a diagnosis.

Many clients need a diagnosis in order to clarify their distress. Having a diagnosis that explains difficulties can provide enormous relief. For example, recognizing that feelings of lethargy, hopelessness, and guilt are part of a depression rather than some ominous character flaw can provide a sense of relief. Once a diagnosis is established, people sometimes think, "Now at least I know what's wrong with me." In addition, a diagnosis generally points the way to an effective treatment approach. Understanding what is wrong allows you to proceed with making it better. Clarifying the problem leads the way to a solution.

It is not a good idea to self-diagnose. The information provided here is to give you an introduction to major diagnostic categories. It takes a skilled clinician to recognize symptoms and differentiate the severity of a characteristic that might warrant intervention. For the beginning student of the mind and diagnosis, the process of categorizing mental distress is perplexing. New students often come to me after talking with a client with a severe diagnosis and say, "There's nothing wrong with that person. They sound just like me." They are unable to identify signs and symptoms because of their empathy. Conversely, after reading about diagnostic categories, many people believe they recognize symptoms in themselves that have been described. They may personalize and misinterpret descriptions.

Mental health symptoms occur on a continuum of normal to pathological, which is why it is sometimes difficult to distinguish between a symptom and an endearing quirk. For example, one symptom of a severe personality disorder is identity disturbance. Most of us experience questions about our identity at one time or another. As we move through developmental and role changes, we wonder anew about our personal identity. This is within the realm of normal. In a person with a character disorder, confusion about role and identity takes on much larger proportions. The person may not be able to choose meaningful work and may move from relationship to relationship in quick succession. The identity disturbance in a client with a severe emotional disorder is a more profound alteration. The normal characteristic is carried to a pathological extreme. So use this introduction as a way to understand how clinicians communicate about psychological disorders. Do not try to fit yourself or people you know into these categories unless you have thoroughly studied diagnostic classification. Bring questions about diagnosis or symptoms to a mental health provider for clarification and discussion.

Clinicians in the United States define diagnosis according to the *Diagnostic & Statistical Manual of Mental Disorders* (DSM) system. The DSM descriptions are developed by a consensus of mental health practitioners from a variety of educational backgrounds. What follows is an introduction to some of the major categories described in the *DSM–IV* (fourth edition).

There are additional categories and diagnoses covered in the manual, such as somatic disorders and conditions related to medical disorders, that will not be discussed here. In addition, keep in mind that there are many systems of diagnostic classification and many ways of understanding diagnoses. This discussion is in no way all-inclusive or complete.

Adjustment Disorder

Many people experience transient, situational emotional distress. When the source of distress can be easily identified and is of a relatively short duration, a person may be diagnosed with an adjustment disorder. For example, if after losing a job someone experiences feelings of depression that last for several weeks or even months, the person may meet criteria for adjustment disorder with depressed mood. Symptoms can be traced back to a specific incident or situation and last for less than six months. Symptoms can include difficulty with emotions or behavior. The person may have anxious or depressed moods or impulsive behaviors.

Treatment of adjustment disorders usually does not require any medications, and the person will respond well to psychotherapy or talking through the issue. When the crisis is resolved, the person may actually function at a higher level, in part because of strength and skills acquired from working through the experience.

Anxiety Disorders

Anxiety is everywhere. For the most part, if we are alive, we are anxious—at least at some level. Human beings are biologically wired for anxiety with a fight or flight response that is psychological and physiological. Anxiety is an energy or tension that exists in a dynamic being. Anxiety is an energy that results from conflicting desires or presses within the mind. Anxiety may be a response to threat or perceived threat. Anxiety provides information about changes that need to occur. It calls our attention to needs that are unmet or dangers in the environment.

Mild anxiety is helpful because it can sharpen our thinking and our senses. Gearing up for a sporting event or a performance can help you use your abilities at peak levels. Moderate anxiety begins to interfere with concentration and can detract from full use of intellectual and emotional faculties. Severe anxiety may immobilize or overwhelm an individual and render them unable to function effectively.

Psychoanalytic concepts of anxiety currently see anxiety as resulting from traumatic situations. According to noted psychoanalyst Charles Brenner in his book, *An Elementary Textbook of Psychoanalysis,* "The psyche is overwhelmed by an influx of stimuli [that] is too great for it either to master or to discharge." Freud saw anxiety as having a biological, genetic basis. He suggested that anxiety helps protect us, and that it can warn us of impending danger. This *signal anxiety* has a useful purpose in terms of promoting our survival. Anxiety becomes a disorder when it interferes with life. The following are some common anxiety disorders.

Generalized Anxiety Disorder involves excessive worrying about several unrealistic concerns for more than two years. For example, a mother may worry about her son failing in high school even though he has straight A's, and worry that the house is dirty even though she cleans it several times each day. This disorder may involve preoccupation, physical tension, and decreased concentration.

Panic Disorder involves discrete episodes of a sudden onset of severe anxiety symptoms, including rapid heart beat, sweating, trembling, nausea, dizziness, fear of going crazy, or fear of dying. By *DSM-IV* criteria, you must have two attacks in a two-week period or at least one attack and fear of having another. Panic Disorder may occur with agoraphobia. Literally translated this means *fear of the marketplace.* It is thought of in layman's terms to mean fear of going outside because clients with this disorder frequently stop leaving their houses. The criteria actually involve fear of being in places from which escape may be impossible or help may be unavailable. It can involve fears of buses, bridges, tunnels, and trains. People with agoraphobia can often leave their house if they have a reliable person to accompany them to assist in case of anxiety or panic.

Specific and social phobias involve fears related to circumscribed stimuli, such as snakes, blood, or public speaking. To be classified as disorders, these fears must interfere with life activities. Although most of us have some specific stimuli we fear, such as heights, injections, or elevators, usually these confere with our lives. Social phobia is characterized by anxiety about being scrutinized. The fear occurs every time the person is faced with the situation. Interestingly, a recent study found that most people are more afraid of public speaking than they are of death. Again, these fears must interfere with daily life before they can be classified as an official disorder.

Obsessive-Compulsive Disorder is characterized by obsessions or recurrent thoughts that are distressing, and compulsions or behaviors designed to neutralize these unpleasant thoughts. The person knows that the thoughts are ridiculous. He also knows that the images or thoughts are coming from his own thoughts. (This is to distinguish between hallucinations and obsessions.) Clients who struggle with Obsessive-Compulsive Disorder are generally in a great deal of distress. The images, thoughts, or impulses are distressing because they often involve violent or sexual content. The behaviors designed to neutralize these thoughts are time-consuming and require constant vigilance. The awareness that thoughts are extreme and behaviors unusual creates a sense of often mortifying shame about symptoms. Clients are anxious because unacceptable thoughts and images interrupt waking consciousness and cannot be easily controlled.

Posttraumatic Stress Disorder was first identified in combat veterans. Clients with this disorder were exposed to a traumatic event that was outside the realm of ordinary life experience, where their physical safety or the safety of others was threatened. The client may experience intrusive recollections, flashbacks, or nightmares about the event. They feel anxious and keyed up, often with an exaggerated startle response. The client may avoid any reminders of the trauma, including people associated with the event and symbols or conversations related to the event.

Anxiety disorders tend to respond well to treatment. Interventions can be used alone or in combination to successfully treat anxiety. Psychodynamic theory suggests that if unconscious conflicts are made conscious, anxiety can be resolved. Pharamcological agents such as Buspar or benzodiazepines can decrease chemical anxiety transmitters. Behavioral interventions such as systematic desensitization and exposure techniques have some success. Obsessive-Compulsive Disorder is tougher to treat but may respond to psychodynamic therapy, or medications such as Anafranil or Luvox. Some treatments for Obsessive-Compulsive Disorder involve behavioral methods such as flooding and response prevention. Posttraumatic Stress Disorder can be treated with interventions that decrease avoidance and help manage anxiety. Symptoms can be managed pharmacologically.

Mood Disorders

Depression is well characterized when Shirley MacLaine as a character in *Steel Magnolias* says, "I'm not depressed. I've just been in a bad mood for forty years." We all experience bad moods. Clinical depression can be distinguished from ordinary depressed feelings in that these moods linger for several weeks. Efforts to resolve these feelings are ineffective.

There are a number of psychodynamic explanations for symptoms of depression. Depression is a natural response to loss. When we lose something important to us—a person, position, or possession—we feel grief. Grief can be seen as a precursor to feelings of depression. Losses of loved ones, from infancy on, produces profound feelings of grief and depression in human beings and animals. Attachment is so important to our survival that there is a universal response to losses of our loved ones.

Depression has been characterized as "anger turned inward." Early on, we learn that anger is an unacceptable emotion. Our Judeo-Christian ethics tell us that anger is sinful, and that we should be forgiving and turn the other cheek. We observe the destructive effects of anger when we see others express these impulses inappropriately. Feedback from parents when we are angry may tell us that it is best not to share these feelings. The tricky part is that we all feel anger. It occurs naturally as a part of emotional life. So what are we to do with these feelings? Often, the mind may direct these energies inward in the form of self-loathing or guilt about even having these thoughts. In other words, depression may result when feelings of anger are turned inward toward the self rather than being outwardly expressed. This mechanism involves a defense against our own aggressive tendencies, which we view as unacceptable and inappropriate.

Depression may also have a biological component. We know that neurotransmitter levels in depressed individuals are different from those of nondepressed individuals. The levels of serotonin and norepinephrine are most often affected. Medications to treat depression can restore these neurotransmitters to more adequate levels and thus produce relief of symptoms.

There are basically two types of mood disorders: unipolar and bipolar. Unipolar depression is characterized by sad, melancholy feelings. Major Depressive Episode involves two weeks of disinterest or depressed mood, often accompanied by changes in sleep, appetite, and energy. There may be thoughts of guilt or suicide. Dysthymia is a more prolonged, moderate level of depression that may have many of the same symptoms as major depression. These types of depression respond well to several forms of treatment, including dynamic and cognitive psychotherapy, and biological interventions such as medications or electroconvulsive therapy.

Bipolar Disorder, or manic depression by its old name, involves both depressed moods and episodes of mania or hypomania. Mania involves an expansive or irritable mood. Hypomania is a slightly less severe manifestation of these symptoms. It may be associated with grandiosity, hypersexuality, excessive involvement in pleasurable activities such as shopping or gambling, and hyperreligiosity. Clients in a manic episode have a decreased need for sleep and may become hyperactive. If allowed to progress, clients will break with reality and become delusional or have hallucinations. The treatment of choice for Bipolar Disorder is psychotherapy and medication. Mood stabilizing medications, including lithium, may be helpful in both treating and preventing symptoms.

Thought Disorders

Schizophrenia is perhaps the most frightening of the disorders because thinking and behaviors are so dramatically different from our own. People with schizophrenia perceive differently and process information differently. These individuals seem so strange because mental functioning is profoundly altered. However, when you are able to understand the language and behavior of schizophrenia, these clients are easily seen as vulnerable rather than scary. Society has difficulty with people who are different. Schizophrenia is viewed by some clinicians as an alternative way of being in the world, rather than just an illness.

Perceptions of reality are altered. Because of impairments in ego functioning, clients may be unable to differentiate between stimuli generated by their own thoughts and those that actually occur in reality. For example, they may hear voices that other people don't hear, and believe them to be real. In schizophrenia, it is as if that part of the mind that is the buffer to the unconscious is defective, and so too much fantasy material leaks into awareness. Life can be full of frightening images of threat and fear and abandonment, distinctly separated from images of joy and goodness. Or the mind may become inactive, impoverished of activity, and dulled both by the effects of the disease and of the drugs used to treat it.

For a long time, we have banished those who are different

to institutions: "out of sight, out of mind." Frequently, people with schizophrenia have spent time in hospitals or mental institutions. This has a profound impact on self-image, even without the mind distortions that accompany a psychotic episode. Since the advent of Thorazine in the 1950s, gradually, people with schizophrenia were returned to the community, with great effort being made to release clients from institutions. New drugs are available to treat the symptoms of schizophrenia, and prognosis today is better than ever. Treatments are more humane, although finding funding for supported community living continues to be a challenge. However, time and again, clients with these altered perceptions have been supported successfully in communities where their differences are understood, accepted, and tolerated. (For more information see R. D. Laing and Thomas Szasz.)

Schizophrenia is characterized by hallucinations and delusions. Hallucinations are altered sensory perceptions, and delusions are fixed false beliefs. In addition, the client may have disorganized speech, disorganized or catatonic behavior, or lack emotional expression, thinking, or constructive planning ability. Clients with this disorder have disturbances in areas of interpersonal relations, work functioning, and/or self-care activities. Continuous symptoms of the disorder must be present for at least six months before a diagnosis can be made. This is because of the seriousness of this particular diagnosis, and the stigma attached to it. We make this diagnosis cautiously.

There are several forms of schizophrenia. The paranoid subtype is characterized by minimal disruption in thinking patterns but preoccupation with threatening delusions or hallucinations. Speech patterns and emotional expressions are not disturbed. This type of schizophrenia tends to become evident between the ages of thirty to forty.

Disorganized Schizophrenia is characterized by speech patterns that are incomprehensible and behavior that is purposeless. Facial expression of emotions may be inappropriate or absent. For example, a client might laugh when talking about something serious. This disorder generally expresses itself in late adolescence or early adulthood.

Catatonic Schizophrenia is relatively rare but is characterized by episodes of catatonic behavior. Catatonic symptoms include a lack of intentional control over movements and decreased physical activity. At times, these clients will sit unmoving for hours. There is a subtype of this diagnosis called Undifferentiated Schizophrenia, which is made for clients with symptoms from several of the other subtypes when one category is not clearly met. Residual Schizophrenia is a classification for clients who continue to have social and vocational symptoms but are not disturbed by active hallucinations or delusions.

Treatment for schizophrenia generally involves medications and increased environmental support during acute episodes. When medications help to control hallucinations and delusions, cognitive behavioral therapy and support of daily living can be useful. Dynamic psychotherapy is not generally used for clients with schizophrenia, because the anxiety that is inherent in that type of therapeutic work might not be tolerable to the client. Therapy should be supportive and geared toward helping the client cope with everyday difficulties. Social-skills training has been shown to have some benefits. Frequently, clients can benefit from supported living arrangements.

Sometimes a person's reality is characterized by delusions or fixed beliefs, but thinking does not involve hallucinations. This is called Delusional Disorder. Examples may be paranoid delusions, such as thinking that someone is out to harm you. Erotomania involves a sexual or romantic preoccupation that is not based in reality. Delusions of grandeur involve an inflated sense of self-esteem.

Personality Disorders

Character can be defined as our enduring personality and patterns. It refers to patterns of feelings, styles of thinking, and patterns of relating. Character disorders are often egosyntonic. In other words, the person with the disorder does not necessarily feel distress. Maladaptive patterns fit with the person's way of thinking or relating. Often, it is those people surrounding the person with the disorder who feel the distress. Many personality disorders develop as a result of developmental difficulties. Personality disorders are pervasive, maladaptive ways of perceiving, relating, feeling, thinking, and behaving. Resolution of these disorders takes time and extended treatment. Change is not superficial but instead involves restructuring character.

Personality disorders are grouped together in three different clusters. Cluster A involves disorders that are characterized by odd or eccentric behaviors. These include Paranoid Personality Disorder, Schizoid Personality Disorder, and Schizotypal Personality Disorder. Cluster B involves disorders that are characterized by dramatic emotions or erratic behaviors. These include Antisocial Personality Disorder, Borderline Personality Disorder, Histrionic Personality Disorder, and Narcissistic Personality Disorder. Cluster C involves disorders that are characterized by anxious and fearful behaviors. These include Avoidant, Dependent, and Obsessive-Compulsive Personality Disorders.

These disorders are an exaggeration of normal aspects of functioning. Because they are related to personality or character, the structure of the disorder is basic to personality, and the effects of symptoms are pervasive in everyday life. These disorders are long term, and their origins are generally found in developmental history and early childhood. *DSM-IV* defines personality disorder as "an enduring pattern of inner experience and behavior" that is different from the usual expectations of a person's culture. Symptoms may affect thinking, emotions, relationships, or impulse control.

Cluster A

Paranoid Personality Disorder This disorder is characterized by pervasive distrust and suspiciousness of others. This person is always worried about being exploited by others and doubts others' loyalty. They see personal attacks everywhere and might harbor grudges.

Schizoid Personality Disorder This person is not interested in personal relationships and does not desire social contact. They have few relationships and prefer solitary activity. They are indifferent to praise or criticism and may be emotionally cold or aloof.

Schizotypal Personality Disorder These clients may be uncomfortable in relationships with others but also experience perceptual alterations and have eccentric behaviors. They may have odd beliefs or magical thinking. Magical thinking is typical of childhood fantasies and fairy tales. For example, believing that if you click your heels three times you will get home. Speech patterns may be odd, as can be emotional expression. Excessive social anxiety might be present.

Cluster B

Antisocial Personality Disorder This disorder is characterized by a tendency to consistently violate the rights of others. These people often have a general disregard for social norms and legal standards. They may lie, cheat, steal, or injure others. They are irresponsible and impulsive. These clients have had emotional difficulties during childhood and meet the criteria for childhood conduct disorder. in severe cases, these individuals frequently end up in jail.

Borderline Personality Disorder This disorder is characterized by unstable interpersonal relationships, an unstable self-image, erratic emotions, and marked impulsiveness. These clients are terrified of abandonment and will go to great lengths to protect themselves from feeling alone. They suddenly move from one intense relationship to the next. They are often unable to select a vocation or career. They may attempt suicide, or injure themselves in physical ways in an attempt to cope with unpleasant feelings. Mood shifts are severe and rapid. These clients struggle with a profound sense of inner emptiness. They may have rage and frequent displays of temper.

Histrionic Personality Disorder Clients with this disorder are excessively emotional and need to be the center of attention. They may be seductive or provocative in their behavior. Their emotions and relationships tend to be shallow.

Narcissistic Personality Disorder These individuals may appear grandiose and self-aggrandizing on the surface, but underneath there is serious difficulty. These clients are compensating for an inner sense of unworthiness, with an outward display of bravado. They may be preoccupied with ideas about their own success and have an excessive need for admiration. They lack the ability for empathy and may be unwilling or unable to understand other people's feelings and perspectives. They may be arrogant or haughty. They have a tendency to see others as being envious of them.

Cluster C

Avoidant Personality Disorder These clients are characterized by social inhibition and feelings of inadequacy.

They are loners but not by choice. They avoid relationships because they are fearful of criticism or being rejected by others. They are reluctant to try new things because they fear being embarrassed.

Dependent Personality Disorder This disorder is characterized by excessive dependency needs or the need to be taken care of by others. This client has difficulty making decisions without consulting with others and tries to avoid responsibilities. They tend to agree with others all the time to avoid conflict. They constantly look for close relationships, and if one person is not available, must look for someone else who can be near. They may be excessively preoccupied with fears about who will care for them if present caretakers become unavailable.

Obsessive-Compulsive Personality Disorder These clients seek order and cleanliness as a way of life. They are consumed by perfectionism and issues of control at the expense of flexibility, openness, and efficiency. They may be preoccupied with details, rules, lists, order, organization, or schedules, to the extent that the point of the activity is lost. They may become obsessed with work-related activities or moral questions. They tend to be rigid, stingy, and stubborn.

We all have character and personality. Some aspects of our character work and are adaptive. Others aspects are not so adaptive. This range or continuum determines whether characteristics are normal or abnormal. Each characteristic that defines a personality disorder can also be found in the range of normal functioning. Certainly it is normal to have dependency and compulsiveness and even some narcissim. Because these disorders are related to degrees of impairment on a continuum, it may be more difficult to diagnose correctly a personality disorder.

Personality disorders are generally treated in longer-term psychotherapies. Dynamic and cognitive-behavioral approaches have been shown to have positive effects. Medications may be used at times to help alleviate serious symptoms.

Addictive Disorders

The effects of addiction are pervasive. We know, work, and live with people who are addicted. We struggle as a society with compulsive wanting. As a nation, we spend huge sums of money attempting to deal with addiction, but as yet we have been largely unsuccessful. Edward Khantzian, a psychoanalyst and addictions psychiatrist at Harvard University, states in his article, "A Contemporary Psychodynamic Approach to Drug Abuse Treatment," "Suffering is at the heart of addictive disorders." We define addiction as the continued use of substances or behaviors despite having knowledge of harmful consequences.

Addiction has multiple causes. Substances have biological properties that stimulate repeated use. Neurochemical actions on the brain at pleasure centers trigger the impulse to use them. Evidence for a genetic component is weak but generally accepted. Behaviors learned from family and peers may influence substance-use patterns. In addition, although we have been unable to identify a single addictive personality, we have been able to identify characteristics that may predispose a personality to express an addiction. For example, clients with difficulty managing anxiety or emotions may find relief, temporarily, in the use of substances. Some addicts say that the first time they felt normal was when they discovered the effects of psychoactive substances. Personality plays a significant role in the establishment and maintenance of addictive patterns.

Addiction is really a heterogeneous set of disorders, with patterns of compulsive use. Substance abuse is characterized by maladaptive patterns of use that interfere with work or other responsibilities, use in situations that are dangerous, legal difficulties, and continued use despite knowledge of damaging consequences. Substance dependence involves these characteristics in addition to development of tolerance and withdrawal symptoms, increasing amounts of time spent in activities related to substance, and unsuccessful attempts to decrease or cut down use.

In addition to the client with the addiction, family members are generally affected by addictive patterns. Family dysfunction may include maladaptive communications, inappropriate expression of anger, violation of boundaries, and the assumption of maladapative roles. Children of substance-dependent clients often assume responsibilities for the family beyond levels that are age-appropriate. They may have to meet parents' physical and financial needs, as well as manage the demands of school, care for younger siblings, and run a household. Spouses of addicted clients develop emotional and psychological difficulties that are complementary to the client. Enabling behaviors and denial are shared ways of relating. Frequently, depression accompanies addiction. There is also a high co-morbidity with personality disorders. The addictive household is unpredictable, often chaotic, and filled with distortions. (For more information, see William Crisman's *The Opposite of Everything is True* and *Bradshaw On: The Family* by John Bradshaw.)

There is reason to be optimistic. Addiction is highly treatable. A number of therapeutic methods is available to support recovery from addiction. Psychotherapy can be combined with pharmacotherapy and fellowship programs.

Eating Disorders

Eating disorders involve severe disturbances in eating patterns. the most common ages for the appearance of eating disorders is late adolescence and young adulthood, ages fifteen to twenty, but they may manifest at anytime during life.

Anorexia and bulimia are the most common eating disorders. These disorders are not just abnormalities of eating patterns but also involve distortions of body perception. Anorexia involves a persistent refusal to maintain minimally normal body weight; an intense fear of gaining weight; and a distorted perception of body size and shape. Bulimia involves patterns of excessive eating and compensatory behaviors to prevent weight gain. The effects of bingeing might be counteracted by abuse of laxatives, exercise, or induced vomiting. Self-evaluation is excessively influenced by a distorted sense of body size and weight. Simple obesity is classified as a medical disorder in the International Classification of Disease (ICD) system, but it is not included in the *DSM-IV* classification system because obesity has not been consistently linked to psychological or psychiatric disorders. However, there is evidence that psychological factors may play a role in some cases of obesity.

Anorexia and bulimia can be serious disorders. Symptoms may recur because of a combination of physiological, psychological, and societal factors. People frequently look to societal factors to explain excessive concern over body shape. While it is true that this society has a narrow definition of what is ideally attractive, societal factors do not explain why one person develops a serious preoccupation with food, while another person can ignore societal pressures and manifest a unique shape and beauty. As with all symptoms, eating-pattern disturbances fall on a continuum. Some people have a mild preoccupation with losing several pounds. This might, in part, be explained by societal expectations and pressures. However, clients who manifest symptoms severe enough to be diagnosed as anorexic or bulimic generally have significant psychological issues and biological involvement.

We learn our eating patterns early in life. Parents focus closely on the eating patterns of their growing children. Indeed, we use weight gain as an indication of developmental progress in infants and children. Optimal child size is linked to optimal parenting and seen as evidence of a thriving child. there may be a link to parental restrictions or control of early eating patterns to some cases of adult eating disorders.

Others suggest that clients with eating disorders are responding to psychological pressures within family relationships, and that they may have an excessive focus on perfection. The client with an eating disorder may feel unable to control many aspects of their emotional life, but they are able to manifest some semblance of perfection in a perfect control of weight or caloric intake. There may be a power struggle at work, as the client asserts control over her food intake rather than allow a parent to define their identity.

Eating disorders are often accompanied by neurochemical changes in the brain. There is some evidence that these brain chemicals and the regions of the brain involved in satiety may contribute to eating disorder symptoms. These symptoms may be tenacious and obsessive in nature. When body-image distortion is severe, the client's thinking may resemble delusional thinking. Certainly, cognitive ideas play a role in the maintenance of these symptoms. For example, a client with an eating disorder may be convinced that life would be perfect if only they could shed that last few pounds. Eating disorder symptoms may occur along with other psychological syndromes, such as with a personality disorder or depression. At times, a psychotic fear of food might lead to restriction of eating.

Depending on the severity of the symptoms, treatment for eating disorders may take time. Clients with anorexia or bulimia may develop physical symptoms that require medical management as a part of the treatment. Electrolyte imbalances and damage to the digestive tract can present life-threatening emergencies. Medications may play a role in restoring neurotransmitter levels. Psychotherapy involves a focus on underlying issues, as well as restoring physical safety through normalizing eating behaviors.

Organic Disorders

The physical and physiological structure of our brain determine, to a large extent, the types and range of thinking and behavior available to the human system. The brain is the physical mechanism that allows for the expression of personality. The brain provides a physical context for mind and is the biological underpinning of behavior. Brain functioning is still poorly understood, as the brain-behavior relationship is only just beginning to be explored.

Damage or injury to any area of the brain will disrupt thinking abilities and alter behavior. These insults to brain tissue may be congenital, or received at or before birth. Injury may occur later in life as a result of trauma, metabolic alterations, or toxins. Deterioration as a result of age may occur. Injury may involve tissue, blood supply, or nerve connections. Changes in production and availability of neurotransmitters may occur as a result of metabolic disturbances. Genetic vulnerability may predispose some individuals to changes in brain functioning.

Dementia is characterized by disturbances in memory. There are several types of dementia, and a number of suspected causes. The most often discussed type of dementia is the Alzheimer's type. This is thought to be due to changes in brain tissue and may have some genetic link. Other causes of dementia include multiple ministrokes, or multi-infarct dementia, also infection from viruses, including HIV or Creutzfeld-Jakob Disease (CJD) syndromes. One case of dementia may have multiple underlying causes.

Seizures are abnormal electrical activity of the brain and may have an impact on behavior or personality. The most common personality effect from seizures is a disorder called Temporal Lobe Epilepsy. Seizure activity in the temporal lobe may cause explosive emotional outbursts. If someone has abrupt onset of anger or aggression, irritability, or impulsive

ating, a diagnosis of Temporal Lobe Epilepsy should be considered.

Brain injury can occur through trauma, vascular accident, or metabolic changes. In rare cases, infection may be responsible for brain injury. Treatment for organic conditions might be rehabilitative and attempt to help the client find ways to compensate with functional loss. Medications may play a role in restoring neurochemical functions. Surgery may be able to correct some structural deficits. (For more information see *The Man Who Mistook His Wife For a Hat,* by Oliver Sacks.)

Where Do I Fit In?

People rarely fit neatly into these diagnostic categories. There may be symptoms of depression, addiction, and a personality disorder, along with organic changes. We are complex beings. We have unique patterns of strengths and limitations. Our biological potential influences our experiences. Our experiences shape our character. Situations influence how we feel and act. The diagnostic classification system looks at general descriptions of symptoms and behaviors. It cannot capture the nuances of individual personality.

For additional information see the *Diagnostic and Statistical Manual of Mental Disorders,* American Psychiatric Association, Washington, D.C., Fourth Edition, 1994.

CHAPTER 4

Getting
Started

People often approach me with questions about psychotherapy or mental health symptoms. They say, "I have a friend who . . . ," or describe a situation and ask if I think it's "normal." Questions about *friends* are frequently about themselves; *someone* is often *me*. My answer to their questions is usually, "What makes you ask" and "Tell me more." Recently a colleague asked, "Do you think Prozac will help someone having a crisis with depression?"

When I offered my standard reply, my colleague Julian described a friend experiencing long-standing feelings of depression, punctuated by episodes of deep despair. I replied that medications may be helpful with this situation but that an ongoing psychotherapy might also be needed. Julian revealed that *he* was the one struggling with feelings of despair and hopelessness.

Once a person recognizes that there is a psychological problem, knowing how or where to get help can be somewhat challenging. Although the process of finding a good match in a therapist can be uneventful, more typically, it requires significant effort. Sometimes the first therapist you call will be compatible, qualified, and available. For other people, the search can be more complicated. Julian's story illustrates the sometimes frustrating process of getting help for emotional difficulties.

If you have tried to find a therapist yourself, some of what Julian encountered might sound familiar. Other aspects of his journey are unique to his particular situation. Finding a therapist who is well suited to you requires persistence, tenacity, assertiveness, and a measure of faith. Good help is available. Keep looking until you find it.

Julian is the type of person who does not like to burden others with his troubles. At work, he focuses on the task at hand and although he is sociable, he does not talk freely about personal problems. So when he approached me with this question about depression, I was aware that his need for help was serious. Before they ask for help most people will try to solve their problems on their own. By the time they ask for help, their own resources are depleted.

I offered Julian the names of several competent local clinicians whom I knew had time available for treatment. Julian set up an appointment for an initial consultation with a well-known, well-respected psychodynamic psychologist. Although Julian told me he felt better after this initial visit, the stresses that were contributing to his depression continued to build in his personal life. Several days after the initial meeting with his therapist, Julian attempted suicide by taking a potentially lethal overdose of cardiac medications. It is not uncommon for people to come into treatment at a time when they feel utterly trapped and without options.

Much to his disappointment, Julian survived his suicide attempt. When he woke up the next morning, he confided in several family members what he had done. Although he had survived the immediate effects of the overdose, Julian decided, at the urging of his family, to seek medical treatment for any lingering aftereffects of the medications. Julian had standard HMO insurance coverage, and was directed by the 1-800 number on his card to seek an evaluation at a local emergency room. The physicians at the ER suggested monitoring Julian's cardiac condition for twenty-four hours despite the absence of any apparent symptoms. Julian told the emergency room staff about his feelings of depression and the details of trying to take his own life. Because of this, a psychiatric consult was requested by the emergency room physician. After twenty-four hours of waiting and repeated requests that the consult be completed, a psychiatrist was still nowhere to be found. It was, after all, Sunday. The psychiatrist on call simply couldn't be reached. When he was medically stable, Julian agreed with the treating physician to leave the hospital rather than wait any longer for a psychiatrist, and to follow up with his depression as an outpatient. The insurance company made a referral to a participating mental health provider, which offered Julian an appointment for an intake in two weeks.

Julian called to tell me what had been happening and asked my advice about both the depression and his wishes to die. He was significantly disappointed at having survived his attempt. He described a messy divorce in process and feelings of extreme anger toward his wife. I urged him to contact the HMO referral service and explain the urgent nature of the situation and request an earlier appointment. They were able to speed up the waiting time and give him an appointment in ten days. In the interim, I suggested he continue to see the psychologist who did the initial evaluation. Although my friend had some reservations about this therapist, he did complete several additional visits with her. In the end, he felt she was too expensive and situated too far from his home. Perhaps of a more serious concern, he did not feel this therapist was supportive enough. Although the work with this therapist was not long term, these meetings did help Julian wait the ten days until an intake could occur through the HMO clinic.

At the clinic a psychiatrist completed an evaluation and

prescribed medications. Julian was assigned to a therapist. These visits were fully covered by insurance. It quickly became apparent that the therapist, although capable of offering support and encouragement, was not qualified to provide in-depth psychotherapy for serious emotional difficulties. The clinic's psychiatrist agreed that a psychodynamic psychotherapy was indicated but recognized that this service was not available through the insurance plan. Julian would need to pay for this out of his own picket. Recognizing that this type of treatment offered the best chances for success, Julian contacted a therapist recommended by the clinic psychiatrist. The new therapist was a prominent, psychoanalytically trained psychiatrist with distinguished credentials. In addition, she had a warm, supportive, interpersonal style and had an office in a nearby area. Finally, Julian was able to engage fully in a treatment process and made a solid, ongoing connection with a qualified treatment provider. I am delighted to report that six months later, therapy is progressing well and suicide is no longer a concern. In fact, Julian has achieved significant relief of his symptoms and has begun a journey of self-exploration that is both enlightening and productive. When asked about treatment, he states, "I'm discovering more than I ever anticipated. For the first time, I'm meeting me! I am honestly surprised at how differently I can feel!"

Finding a qualified therapist who matches both your needs and style may take some work. Keep at it. Ask questions. State your preferences. Tell prospective therapists your likes and dislikes. Talk to friends. Ask your insurance representative for providers they use, but don't limit your search because of insurance reimbursement patterns. If you meet with a therapist who rubs you the wrong way, don't be afraid to make a change. Look for a therapist the same way you would search for a cardiac surgeon or an oncologist. At stake is your mind, your mental health, and sometimes, as for Julian, your life. In the end, finding a therapist who is qualified and compatible will be well worth the effort.

Why People Go for Treatment

The decision to seek professional counseling often comes at a time of overwhelming distress or confusion. People seek help when the pain they feel outweighs their fears about asking for professional assistance. The idea to get help may be our own, or the suggestion of someone who is close to us. Sometimes we realize on our own that we need to talk over our problems with someone we can trust. At other times, people around us—either family or coworkers—might notice signs of distress and suggest getting some help. Whether concerns arise from within us or from the feedback of others, if the idea of seeking counseling keeps coming up, it may be worth investigating the possibilities.

When we seek treatment is influenced by the value we place on psychological matters, our confidence in treatment, availability and cost of consultation, and our acceptance of emotional difficulties. Perhaps the most important factor in motivating someone to seek treatment is their level of distress. When we feel a great deal of emotional pain, or unresolved psychological distress, we are more likely to set aside any fears we might have about admitting we need help, and get it. When the pain outweighs the fear of coming for treatment and treatment can offer even the slightest glimmer of hope, we will make that first, deep-breath call.

Some people have an idea about what is causing their distress. Others are simply aware of vaguely feeling "bad." Still others have a sense that something just isn't right, without having a clear idea about what is contributing to their problem. Sometimes we have misconceptions about what is causing symptoms. For example, someone might blame others for recurrent difficulties when the problem really is some aspect of themselves. Other people may blame themselves for difficulties or feel guilty about causing a problem, when they are not really responsible for the situation. For example, a client who is depressed may blame themselves for these feelings. They may even begin to believe "I am a depressed person" or "I'm not a good human being because I can't appreciate happiness every day." They may feel defective because they feel depressed. In reality, the person may have good reasons to be angry about situational factors. Feelings of depression can indicate that there is a problem based in reality and that real life changes need to occur.

Our beliefs about the mind-body relationship will influence the type of treatment we seek. Some people believe that emotional distress is the result of a biological cause and look for treatment that involves biological interventions. Although some symptoms are primarily biological in nature, psychological distress generally has multiple underlying causes. In other words, symptoms are multidetermined and result from a matrix of contributing factors. Thoughts, feelings, relationships, real-life situations, and unconscious forces may all contribute to and interact with biology to create and sustain a particular symptom.

When we see mind and body as interconnected and interdependent, we devote equal attention to physical and mental health. Can you imagine a health-care system that encourages regular emotional checkups and preventive psychological care in equal measure with physical medical care? In addition to our family physician, we might even arrange for a family psychologist to assess development, prescribe prevention activities, and monitor emerging symptoms or difficulties.

As a society we sometimes have a tendency to adopt a

pull-yourself-up-by-the-bootstraps attitude toward emotional problems. Some of our cultural values have influenced us to see emotional distress as unimportant or willful laziness, or in extreme cases, as evidence of sinfulness. For example, when someone has not experienced clinical depression, it is difficult to understand why a person cannot simply shake off or overcome feelings of depression. Ordinary sadness passes, so why not depression? In addition, perhaps we fear the symptoms we observe in seriously mentally ill clients. We might be ashamed to admit that we have felt some of these symptoms too, and fear being compared with them, or labeled as crazy.

Our view on psychology or psychiatry are shaped by personal experiences, culture, and ethnic background, as well as the media and the advice of people we respect. If we view mental health professionals as highly educated scientific care givers, we may interact with them as we do our medical providers. On the other hand, if we believe psychotherapy only provides useful fodder for situation comedies, we are unlikely to discuss serious problems with people we see as comedians.

We have learned about therapy from Hollywood, as well as the medical system. Our views on the benefits of psychotherapy have been influenced by Woody Allen, Bob Newhart, and Frazier. We have seen Hollywood versions of in-patient treatment in moves such as *One Flew Over the Cuckoo's Nest, Frances,* and *The Snake Pit.* Many specific disorders have been dramatized in films such as *Ordinary People, Nuts, What About Bob?,* and *The Fisher King.* News coverage offers information about mental health and has an impact on how we view seeking treatment. When a public figure becomes open about some personal psychological issue, our acceptance of the difficulty may increase. For example, when Betty Ford publicly announced her struggle with addiction, it contributed to a decreasing stigma associated with addiction. When Ronald Reagan announced that he was struggling with memory difficulty, our interest in working effectively with these symptoms was heightened.

Reasons for Not Seeking Treatment

It is always interesting to see why some people decide not to seek treatment, even in the face of significant distress. Some people have a natural tendency to see problems as belonging to others. Others believe psychotherapy has no relevance for them but is instead for people with mental illness.

Women seek treatment more often than men. Gender has an effect on how likely we are to express our feelings, and how willing we are to be in the dependent position of admitting a need for help. Historically, women have been encouraged to focus on and express their emotional responses, which is why they are more likely to call attention to any psychological distress they might be experiencing and to be referred for treatment more often. Men see themselves as self-sufficient and have traditionally been reluctant to admit needing support from others.

It has been my experience that the healthiest person in a family system often seeks treatment first. Admitting that there is a problem and asking for support in looking for a resolution takes relative amounts of personality strength. Having the courage to address difficulties inherently implies a healthy ability for introspection. Conversely, the clients who are most fragile may need some coaxing to enter into consultation.

It is important to understand that the person who says, "I don't have any problems" or "I don't need any help" may be doing so out of fear and anxiety. Having the strength to say "Maybe it is me" or "Sure, I could use some support" is difficult if you feel ashamed or at fault. Because many of us have been judged harshly during our developmental years, we develop a tendency to judge ourselves harshly. This shame may keep us from feeling able to freely discuss concerns with a therapist. The fear of being criticized may keep some people away from treatment.

At times, clients may be afraid of losing control of impulses with a therapist. For example, someone who struggles with anger may fear that talking about it may increase the problem. Someone who fears their neediness may be reluctant to burden a therapist. These clients can be helped to see that talking about feelings generally leads to less acting out of these impulses. The therapist can be relied on to give feedback about what is appropriate behavior.

Frankly, cost is an issue for most clients. Few people have discretionary income that can easily be devoted to medical expenses. The choice to have therapy often means a commitment of finances, which places a value on the process and ensures that it will not be undertaken casually. If therapy were offered free of charge, we might more readily seek counsel. However, because we do generally have to pay for the process, we may be more diligent about using therapy to its utmost potential.

Fears of Being Judged

Clients frequently fear that therapists will be judgmental. This fear of being judged may interfere with seeking treatment. In sessions, clients often confess actions or thoughts they feel guilty about, and then wait for the therapist's negative reaction. Even though it is common knowledge that therapists are supposed to be nonjudgmental, clients fear that we are secretly labeling their disclosure as acceptable or unacceptable. In general, a therapist will only offer a judgment if there is some risk of harm to a client or another. For example, most therapists would probably state a direct opinion about behavior that is actually destructive in nature. Other than that, most therapists take a nonjudgmental stance on any thoughts or feelings. They are considered grist for the mill, and something to be worked with, not a reason to condemn the client. Therapists are exposed to a wide experience of human nature, and encounter thoughts and feelings that are diverse, complex, and intense.

Clients sometimes accuse me of being secretly and personally judgmental despite my obvious neutral attitude and willingness to explore. One client suggests, "I know you're supposed to be neutral as a psychologist and all, but don't you think (so and so behavior) is crazy?" We might wonder about the client's eagerness to have the therapist judge their behaviors. In invoking early parental relationships, the client gives illusionary power to the therapist, believing he has the ability to know what is right and wrong for the client. It is a wish, a fantasy that the therapist can tell them what to do. The therapist is no more able to give approval than any other human being. Therapists are mere mortals. I have learned through my clinical experiences that knowing what *should* happen is not possible. We cannot know what should have happened and in most cases do not have the wisdom to judge something as right or wrong. For example, a client might ask, "Was I wrong to have had that argument?" How can we know? The argument happened. It is to be understood and the client should learn from it.

Now that I have told you about how therapists are nonjudgmental, let me tell you how we are judgmental. Therapists make judgments about symptoms. Therapists learn to recognize conditions identified in diagnostic systems. They learn to recognize symptom severity by working with many different clients. Therapists learn to make distinctions between coping mechanisms and use of defenses. This type of judgment is made in order to facilitate the development and well-being of the client. The therapist's judgments are not intended as criticism.

Therapists will make judgments about behaviors that involve injury to yourself or another. This includes forms of sexual or physical abuse. Therapists can help you to see boundary violations and should be able to help you reality-test what is hurtful and what is helpful. When I say to a client who has been sexually abused, "That should not have happened to you," I am making a judgment. If a client is using substances destructively or violating another person's rights, I will tell them I think it is harmful. Rather than seeing this as being judgmental, it should be viewed as the therapist lending a healthy perspective on reality.

Finding a Therapist

Finding a therapist is no easy task. In many cases, when one is looking for a therapist, there is some problem that may leave a person vulnerable to promises of relief. Emotions may be raw or thinking distorted, making rational choices about care providers more difficult.

Most people begin the search for a therapist in the yellow pages, which is perhaps the worst way to find one. These ads are marketing tools and offer little information about interpersonal or clinical skills. If you must use this information, do so to generate a list of names, and call for more information about available treatment. Talk with the therapist on the phone to evaluate interpersonal skills.

Perhaps the most useful method of introduction is a friend's recommendation. Someone who personally has had experiences with the therapist will be a better judge of interpersonal or clinical functioning. However, if you are referred through a personal contact, reimbursement for treatment through a third-party payor may be less likely. Insurance companies tend to work with closed networks of providers. If you do decide to use someone who is highly recommended but out of the network, you can expect to pay out of pocket for this type of arrangement. Negotiate a price that is affordable in the long run. Plan to budget an ongoing amount for therapy expenses. Therapists generally will reduce fees to a certain extent and are encouraged to work *pro bono* in some cases. If you cannot afford the full fee, look for a therapist willing to arrange low-fee services.

In many cases, referral to a mental health provider can be obtained from a primary medical care provider or through an insurance company. When prior approval is obtained from a managed-care network, many companies will pay for ten to thirty sessions per year with an approved provider. If you are seen in a group-practice setting, be sure to ask for credentials of your therapist.

Names of therapists can also be obtained from professional organizations: American Psychological Association, American Psychiatric Association, American Psychoanalytic Association, state medical societies, and licensing boards. Keep in mind that these services are not endorsing specific therapists but are only referring to them. The local universities may offer a source of recommendations. Call the department of graduate psychology or medical schools and ask about clinicians in the area. Many teaching institutions run low-fee clinics with bright, motivated students as staff.

Your Expectations

What you expect to get from therapy has an impact on whether or not you will actually seek it. When we become aware of emotional difficulties, or disequilibrium, we weigh the risks and benefits of starting therapy. On the positive side is the potential for relief of symptoms and the hope of psychological support. If we have known people who have benefited from the process of therapy, we may want these benefits for ourselves. Some of the negative aspects of seeking treatment include cost, time, and emotional effort, as well as the inevitable fear of change.

It is reasonable to expect a therapist to establish regular private appointment times, and to keep them. It is reasonable to expect a therapist to listen attentively and carefully to your concerns and offer comments or feedback that will be useful in resolving your difficulties. It is reasonable that the therapist will establish a mutually acceptable fee for services. It is also reasonable for you and your therapist to discuss the goals of the treatment and design a method of approaching the resolution.

Unreasonably high expectations about therapy present as much difficulty as expectations that are too low. If you believe that therapy will produce consistent happiness, or that you can be completely cured of what ails you, you are likely to be disappointed. Therapy cannot produce everlasting happiness. It is impossible to *finish* self-development and self-exploration. As has been noted, therapy can transform misery into common ordinary unhappiness, which is quite an accomplishment when you think about it. But it is certainly true that life after therapy continues to contain challenge, heartache, anxiety, and sadness.

When a client has unrealistically low expectations of the treatment process, they may be unlikely to engage fully in the process. Ideas such as "this will never work" or "shrinks can't help" might impair the motivation for continuing in treatment. These attitudes minimize the positive results that therapeutic work can yield. Generally, clients who participate in the therapy process are satisfied. They see positive effects even if the contact is somewhat limited. Studies in general show a positive effect in clients who do participate in therapy versus clients who do nothing about their problems.

The Deep-Breath Phone Call

Once you have selected several names, it is time to make contact. Many people feel anxious at this point and may hesitate. They may think, "Well, it's not really that bad a problem," or that the therapist will think their concerns are silly or too small to warrant discussion. Take a deep breath, set aside your fears, and make the call anyway. Just think of it as a way to obtain information.

Here is an imaginary scenario of how the process of the first phone contact might go: You sit anxiously by the phone, hesitating and at the same time eager to make the call. You look at your list. Dr. Sally Smith. You think, "sounds unpretentious, down to earth." You dial her number, and a harsh voice comes on a static-filled answering machine asking you to leave your name and number. You get nervous and don't particularly like her tone, so you hang up. You move down to the next name on the list. This therapist's machine has a warm, welcoming message and reassures you that your call is important and that he will get back to you by the end of the working day. You leave your name, number, and when you can be reached, and perhaps a brief description of why you are calling. "I'm interested in a consultation for psychotherapy. If you have been referred by someone the therapist may know, leave that information, too. The third place you call has a receptionist who asks you what the problem is and what insurance coverage you have. The receptionist offers an appointment next Thursday. When you ask to speak with the prospective therapist, she tells you it's not procedure but that one will call you back as soon as they are available. So, now you have taken the first step. Contact has been made. Relax, take a deep breath, and then wait.

Several things can happen on the return call. Ideally, the doctor with the warm, welcoming message will call back later that day. His manner on the phone puts you at ease, and you are able to tell him a bit about why you are interested in treatment. You can ask some questions about the types of treatment offered and times he has available. Ask also if he has a sliding-fee scale, and what fee can be expected for the initial consultation. If all goes well, you set up an appointment. (Don't forget to get directions to the office.)

One client experienced a first contact similar to this—with one snag: The therapist was about to go on vacation and could not start therapy right away. The client decided that working with this therapist was worth the wait and managed his difficulties with the help of friends for that month; he began intensive psychotherapy when the therapist returned.

Return phone calls might not go so well. Imagine this scenario: The therapist from the clinic returns your call two days later. She is courteous but somewhat guarded. She asks how she can help you, but when you ask her to describe the type of treatment she practices, she explains that this will happen on the intake. She is vague about how she works with clients and becomes defensive when you ask her about her qualifications. During the call you are vaguely aware of feeling uncomfortable. If this is the case, it may be best to decline politely any appointments and continue your search by expanding your list of potential therapists; make more calls.

Sometimes finding a good therapist takes one phone call. Sometimes it takes fifteen. Don't be afraid to interview prospective therapists about the type of treatment offered, their qualifications for practice, their educational preparation, and their standard fees. Ask about areas of expertise and what types of difficulties they work with most frequently. The phone contact process should offer your first opportunity to build a trusting rapport with a new therapist. If a therapist is uncomfortable with the process, becomes defensive, or doesn't have time for this brief conversation, it may be difficult to work with them in the future.

Your First Visit

No matter how experienced you are with psychotherapy, the first meeting with a new therapist will create some anxiety. If you expect it, you can take steps to minimize it by using relaxation techniques and preparing for the initial visit. If you are particularly confident in new situations, you may wish to think of general topics you want to cover. If you tend to be more nervous, write a list of things you wish to discuss.

First impressions are important. Is the office setting professional? Do the acoustics allows conversations to remain private? Is the therapist likable and professional? Did you feel comfortable at that first handshake? Do you become more at ease as you begin to discuss your concerns?

A typical first interview begins with introductions. The therapist may ask how you were referred and what brings you for counseling. This is an invitation for you to describe, in your own words, the concerns that prompted you to seek therapy. Feel free to describe your concerns honestly, disclosing information you feel is important to the therapist. As you describe your concerns, you will undoubtedly be watching the therapist's responses. Are they listening, perhaps taking notes? Are they asking questions to elicit details? Does the therapist let you talk without interrupting? Does he ask questions that lead to discovering important details about the current situation?

The focus of the first session should generally be on your current concerns. Whatever *you* see as the *main issue* should take up a significant amount of time in the first session. In addition to your concerns, therapists will want to understand the difficulty in a context, so they will have questions of their own. Therapists may guide the interview to address questions such as: What are the major symptoms? When did it start? Are symptoms periodic or continuous? How severe are symptoms? What makes the symptoms better? Has this ever happened before? Are you taking any medications? Do you have any physical/medical problems? Have you ever been hospitalized? Operated on? What other treatments have your tried? (See table 4-1 for help in preparing for the first meeting.)

| Table 4-1 | **Preparing for the First Visit** |

Take time before your first appointment to reflect on these questions:

What is the main problem?

What other areas do you want addressed?

What do you think contributed to the current difficulties? How do you understand the problems you want addressed?

Is there anything in your personal or family history that you think might be contributing to your current concern?

What are your goals for therapy? What are you hoping for?

What type of treatment are you interested in?

Are there any types of treatment to which you are opposed?

How much money are you willing to put toward treatment if it is not covered by insurance?

What time can you make available for therapy appointments?

It is also helpful to have a history about your early life as well as your current situation. Your therapist will want to know about any previous emotional difficulties. Keep in mind that standard time allowed for an initial appointment is forty-five to sixty minutes. Therefore, some clinicians will recommend scheduling several appointments for an extended evaluation. This allows for a thorough examination of the difficulties and enables client and therapist to work together to form a workable treatment plan.

On the first visit—in addition to getting to know you, building trust, and assessing whether you like the therapist—there are also many tasks to complete. Here is a checklist to help organize your approach to the first session:

_____ Ask the therapist about their education credentials

_____ Establish a schedule for the initial evaluation process

_____ Establish a fee that is mutually acceptable

_____ Exchange phone numbers, and discuss methods of communication if needed

_____ Discuss the limits of confidentiality

_____ Discuss the need for medical/physical evaluation, or needed lab tests

(See also Tables 4-2 and 4-3 for more help in evaluating prospective therapists.)

In addition to these tasks, during your first meeting with the therapist you are deciding if you can trust him. You are evaluating interpersonally and assessing how the therapist reacts to emotions, anger, boundaries, and subjects you consider to be taboo. There are endless ways to see if the therapist is trustworthy, and it is important that you evaluate and form an opinion. Most clients rapidly develop a sense of the competence or incompetence of a therapist. If a therapist makes suggestions that don't work, their credibility is suspect. If a therapist lends observations that clarify situations and facilitate resolutions through new perspectives, a sense of trustworthiness is developed.

Trust is also developed through the therapist's responsible actions. If a therapist is on time for appointments, ready to

| Table 4-2 | **Initial-Visit Interview Guide** |

Here are some questions you might think about asking your potential therapist on your first visit. (If you are seeing a therapist in a group practice for an initial visit, clarify if the person doing the intake is the therapist you will be working with on an ongoing basis.)

1. Where did you go to school?

2. What is the highest degree you obtained, and in what field of study?

3. What is your approach to therapy? What types of treatment do you use?

4. What licenses to practice do you hold? Have you ever lost your license to practice?

5. Where have you worked in the past?

6. What are your areas of expertise?

7. What type of patients do you prefer to work with?

8. What type of patients do you least like to work with?

9. Are you taking new clients at this time? What times are available for regularly scheduled meetings?

10. What is your usual fee? How do you work with insurance? If I cannot afford your usual fee, do you work on a sliding-scale fee?

work at the appointed time, and cancels appointments only in the most serious of emergencies, the therapist communicates through his behaviors that he is trustworthy. Behavior communicates, "I am here when I say I am going to be here." There is also a strong message that the therapist will be reliable, as long as the work continues.

Emotional impressions are important. If it is possible to work successfully with a therapist, you will know early on after several sessions. It is important that the therapist and client agree that working successfully together is possible. This is called a therapeutic alliance. The beginnings of the therapeutic alliance are created in the first session.

If during your first meeting you are not comfortable with the therapist, it is important to say so and express as directly

Table 4-3 | **First Impressions**

After your initial appointments, take time to reflect on the following questions as you evaluate whether this therapist is a good match for you:

Did you like the therapist? Was the therapist warm but professional?

Was the therapist nonjudgmental?

Were you treated with respect and courtesy?

Did the therapist seem comfortable answering questions about credentials and qualifications, without becoming defensive?

Did you feel supported?

Did you feel the therapist was genuinely interested in what you had to say?

Did you feel free to speak your mind?

Did you feel free to disagree with the therapist?

Did the therapist have a positive attitude?

Did the therapist seem to take problems in stride, optimistic about finding solutions and improving your situation?

Did the therapist listen without interrupting?

Was the therapist able to keep the focus on your concerns?

Did you have a sense that the therapist actually understood what you were communicating?

Were there times when the therapist seemed to pay attention to the things you did not say, as well as what you did say? In other words, was the therapist able to explore areas that did not necessarily come to your mind?

Did your goals for treatment seem to be in concert with the therapist's goals? Were you able to plan a mutually agreeable approach toward meeting these goals?

Did the therapist talk to you in words you could understand, without using jargon?

Are fees reasonable?

Does the therapist have provisions for emergency situations?

as you can what is making you uncomfortable. If the matter cannot be resolved to your satisfaction, it is probably best to try to meet with several other therapists. Don't stay with a therapist if from the beginning he makes you feel uncomfortable. At anytime during therapy, if a therapist is demeaning or verbally abusive, wants to touch you, or spends a great deal of time talking about themselves, you should consider another therapist, as these are inappropriate to good therapeutic work and will interfere with your progress.

Evaluating a Therapist

Do you feel comfortable with this person? Is she attentive without being intrusive? Can you talk openly and freely? Ask about areas of concentration or specialty. Are fees reasonable? Does the therapist listen and seriously consider what you're saying?

You don't want a therapist who talks about themselves. The focus of the work in therapy is you. You should not be spending time during the session talking about the therapist's problems. If this happens, address it directly, and ask her to focus on your concerns. If she can't keep the focus on you, change therapists.

Avoid a therapist who dismisses your concerns or is abrupt in interactions. This may seem an unnecessary concern. How could a psychiatrist or psychologist be such a poor communicator? Well, I'm sorry to say, it happens. I have seen providers who performed rote examinations rather than talking with clients. Clinicians can be rushed by insurance-company paperwork and fire off questions at a client, putting off the client's presenting concerns. If a psychotherapist treats you rudely, does not make eye contact with you when listening, or does not appear interested, ask for another therapist. If your therapist patronizes you or minimizes your concerns, get another opinion.

Nobody's Perfect

There are no perfect therapists. Every therapist brings strengths and limitations to the treatment process. The therapist's formal education and personal awareness will impact their treatment style. The client's needs and style will have a greater or lesser fit with the range of therapeutic resources available from a particular therapist. An ideal match between therapist and client will be good enough to achieve the goals of the therapy. A good enough therapist will be able to help you reach your desired goals. A good-enough therapist can recognize and admit mistakes that inevitably occur during the course of a human interaction such as therapy. The good-enough therapist is genuine and therefore fallible. A good-enough therapist need not have invented a theory to implement it effectively. A good-enough therapist makes mistakes but can admit it. Honesty, not brilliance, is necessary for the process of psychotherapy.

In addition, the process of psychotherapy itself may be as important, if not more important, than the therapist's skills and qualities. The very act of talking to another human being about concerns can stimulate change or produce insight. As long as the therapist doesn't interfere with the natural process, the client is likely to make some headway. Some clients will talk through to solutions regardless of what contribution the therapist makes. Other clients will be unable to use information given by skilled or highly qualified therapists.

Evaluating a Therapy

Because progress in therapy may be uneven or uncomfortable, it is often difficult to determine how well things are going. Are goals being met? Is progress being made toward identified goals? It is a good idea to periodically stop to review progress with the therapist. In any ongoing therapy, there will be times of rapid growth and plateaus where little appears to be changing. Staying the course during the plateaus can set the stage for future development and insight. Therapy may remind us of the Zen story about the monk who is walking in the woods one day, gets hit in the head with a pebble, and suddenly achieves enlightenment. It is tempting to say the pebble created the enlightenment. However, it was the thirty years of daily walks and meditation in the woods that readied the monk to be enlightened at the moment the pebble hit.

CHAPTER 5

Structure, Form, and Content

Structure

Therapy comes in many structures or forms: two people, three people, groups of related people, groups of unrelated people, even communities can get together for therapy. *One* person can go to therapy alone and will focus with the therapist on individual issues. *Couples* may go for counseling to work on relationship or marital concerns. *Families* might attend together in order to improve communication styles and learn more problem-solving skills. *Groups* of people with common issues may come together for support, or to collaborate on information sharing, or problem solving. Each structural type of therapy has strengths and limitations that are unique to that structure.

The nature of the therapy structure will be determined to some extent by the number of participants, as well as the number of therapists involved. Who actually attends the sessions will have an impact. The personality styles of individual members will contribute to the unique characteristics of the dyad or group involved in the therapeutic work. The goals that participants bring to the therapy sessions will help to identify which type of structure should be used.

Some characteristics of therapy will be common to all forms. The need for trust and confidentiality are basic to any therapy. Safety to explore issues and discuss thoughts and feelings is necessary for any therapy to proceed. Other characteristics will vary across forms of therapy. The role of the therapist may be different from setting to setting. In individual treatment the relationship between therapist and client may be intense because of the one-on-one interactions. In group therapy, relationships between group members may be quite strong. Group therapy generally does not involve contact between members outside the group setting. Family therapy may involve increased activity among participants and homework assignments from the therapist. Family members are expected to interact between sessions, to observe interactions, and to practice new behaviors.

Individual Therapy

So . . . you are considering individual psychotherapy. Individual therapy is the most common form of psychotherapy. Individual treatment involves private consultation with a therapist. A therapist and a client meet alone, behind closed doors. Individual therapy offers a relationship that involves the unique experience of being fully attended to and understood in a nonjudgmental way by another human being. Meeting with a therapist alone allows for the greatest amount of privacy. Privacy lays the foundation for trust. Trust makes it possible to talk honestly about life's experiences and concerns.

The therapist in individual therapy functions as a balanced participant-observer. The relationship offers support and collaboration on identified problems. Individual therapy allows for a highly personalized treatment plan and individualized attention. Communications can be tailored to match your unique emotional and intellectual style.

Individual psychotherapy allows for the greatest intensity of attention between client and therapist. When treatment goes on over time, a deep relationship is often formed. The transference that develops is most intense in individual treatment and allows for maximum understanding of the process of projection. (Transference will be discussed in detail later, however, briefly, it is the remnants of old relationships projected onto the therapist.) Projection is the process of ascribing ideas from within your own thinking onto a person, and not seeing that person as they are. For example, if you believe that all teachers are authoritarian, you will tend to see teachers you encounter as authoritarian. In reality, teachers have a number of different styles: participatory, autocratic, laissez-faire, etc. You may react to these teachers as if they are authoritarian no matter their style. Ideas about people or relationships can find a blank screen in the therapist's neutral positions. When ideas such as these are attributed to the therapist, presumably the therapist is skilled at watching for distortions in how he is being viewed. When the ideas are transferred in a deeply understood relationship, the process of projection becomes conscious. When it is conscious, it will be more easily changed and less likely to interfere with reality.

The real relationship between client and therapist may provide a consistent, predictable form of attention and support. The client may experience a relationship for the first time that is reliable and consistent. As a relationship builds, the context of the therapy allows the client to feel contained. There is a psychological holding that develops within the context of ongoing therapy sessions. The relationship between client and therapist offers a psychological holding environment that helps to contain the client's conflicts and emotions.

Some therapists suggest that the therapy relationship offers a potential for a corrective emotional experience that can heal injuries from previous relationships which may have contained significant deficits. For example, imagine that a client's parents were emotionally unavailable because of the demands of high-pressure careers. The client may have felt neglected as a child and developed wounds to her self-esteem. She may feel unworthy of attention and angry about not getting what she sees is rightly deserved. For the client in therapy as an adult or adolescent, this may be replayed. The client may react to the therapist as if he is unavailable and neglectful. When the therapist is consistent and reliable and the distortion is pointed out, the client comes to see this distortion. At that point, she may see how distortions such as these might operate in other relationships. Change can now occur because of her awareness.

In addition, the therapist's consistent attention may improve the client's sense of self-worth. The process of therapy allows the client to see that her experience is worthy of exploration and attention and that her feelings and thoughts are to be valued. This validation of self-worth can improve emotional adjustment, and is, in part, the result of the actual aspects of attention in psychotherapy.

One drawback to individual treatment may be the cost. Because it requires individual attention, fees paid to clinicians are greater than in other forms of therapy. The time commitment for individual therapy is significant. Generally, sessions take place once or twice a week, for forty-five to fifty minutes. If current responsibilities include work, studies, and family, scheduling this amount of time may seem difficult.

In addition, some clients may not be able to tolerate the anxiety associated with such concentrated attention. Individual therapy can be tough work! It does not allow for escape from focus. Even if the client is quiet, the attention to the process is sustained. This focus may be too intense for a client who is really uncomfortable with close interpersonal relationships. If this is the case, it may be useful for the therapist and client to engage in an activity while talking, such as walking outdoors, or playing pool, cards, or checkers.

Group Therapy

If you are concerned about relationship and interpersonal difficulties, group therapy may be the preferred method of treatment. It may be the treatment of choice for clients with common concerns and issues. For example, someone who is working to resolve issues related to divorce or being widowed might benefit from meeting others in similar situations. Group treatment offers opportunities to work directly on developing relationship skills, with the benefit of immediate feedback from others. Group therapy is generally available at a lower cost than individual therapy, because one therapist can see a number of people simultaneously. Group therapy introduces peers who can offer real support and perspective on common issues. In some cases, it may be helpful for clients of similar levels of adaptation to meet and exchange feedback and support. For example, a group of clients with serious symptoms might meet to focus on common concerns. Or a group of physicians might benefit from meeting together. In other situations, clients with severe levels of mental illness may benefit from group meetings with clients of a more successful level of adaptation. Clients of different levels of adaptation can offer a variety of experiences that might produce positive results.

Therapy in a group may decrease feelings of shame. The very act of sharing with other people can effectively neutralize feelings of shame. Peers can offer feedback from a perspective of shared experiences. In a group, members can say, "I've had that experience, too," while in therapy, the therapist often has not experienced what the client has.

Feedback from peers may be more credible than coming from a therapist who has not experienced the difficulty. For example, this form of therapy has been found to be particularly useful with clients who have substance-abuse difficulties. Addicts are more likely to confront maladaptive behaviors in each other and promote honesty in pursuit of recovery. Sex offenders and spouse abusers may benefit from feedback from peers.

Group therapy may not be the treatment of choice. Group therapy requires that the needs of the group be addressed first, which may not leave enough time to focus on individual concerns and needs. If an individual will not have adequate opportunities to focus on their own issues, group therapy may not be the best format. Clients who have a great deal of shame or guilt may be too nervous to talk in front of others, which might make group work uncomfortable. For example, someone working on concerns about sexuality might be reluctant to discuss these issues in front of others.

Group therapy is sometimes combined with individual work to obtain the benefits of both forms of therapy. An individual therapist may refer a client to a group treatment that is independent from his practice. The therapist will not participate in group treatment but may receive periodic reports from the group therapist. In this case, the client has a greater role in bringing back to individual sessions insights gained in group therapy. However, it is also common for a therapist who practices both individual and group therapy to recommend participation of a client in one of his own groups. The client receives the benefits of group work but also schedules individual sessions to concentrate on personal issues. The group provides support and feedback, and individual meetings allow for deeper exploration.

Therapy groups may be time-limited or ongoing. That is, groups may meet for a set number of sessions established in advance. For example, a group that focuses on recovery from smoking addiction may meet for ten sessions over ten weeks. Or a group may continue as long as members have an interest, or until the group is no longer needed by most members, as members have reached their goals.

Membership in groups may be open or closed. Closed groups identify participating members at the outset, and a commitment is made to see the group work through to its natural closure. Participants who wish to join while the group is in progress are not permitted to do so. Open-membership groups allow for the inclusion and departure of group members. There is a fluid group membership, dependent on the setting and purpose of the group. An example of an open group is frequently found in inpatient settings. Clients are admitted to the group when they are admitted to a unit and will participate for the duration of their hospital stay. Membership may change daily.

Groups that have a stable, consistent membership move through predictable developmental phases. Initially, group work focuses on building trust and allowing members to establish a rapport. During these early meetings, the group may rely on the therapist's participation to facilitate communication. Middle phases of group meetings focus on group work, and reliance on the therapist decreases. As the group approaches its conclusion, issues of termination come to the surface. Group members plan for ongoing personal development and cope with the loss of the support gained from the group.

Group therapy may be structured according to a number of theoretical perspectives. Group-as-a-whole theory looks at the group as a single dynamic entity. Noted University of California psychiatrist Irving Yalom wrote a definitive text on inpatient group therapy, and offers a method for structuring single-session group meetings. He suggests that the beginning of a group meeting involve each participant identifying goals for that particular meeting. The next segment of group work involves individual members sharing their personal concerns. The second half of the meeting involves the therapist weaving common threads together for the group to share. The last few minutes of the meeting involve a wrap-up of what was gained and processed during that particular meeting.

Family Therapy

When it is difficult to identify a single client and the entire family system seems to be in distress, it may be most economic to consider family therapy. For example, if on evaluation it seems that every member of the family could benefit from psychotherapy, it may be cost effective to bring each of these family members in for work together. Factors that are stressing the entire environmental system can be addressed. Family members can improve communication and break maladaptive patterns.

The goal of family therapy is to improve family functioning and thus improve individual family member satisfaction. It is not unusual for a family to present for treatment with one child having been identified as the patient. Children are masters at assisting the family team to achieve its goals. When a child senses conflict between parents, he will express a symptom that drags the family in for help. This generally involves difficulties at school or problems with discipline. It is rare indeed to have a child manifest symptoms that are not a result of their environment. A child's dysfunction is generally a cry for help or a way to bring family difficulties to the attention of care providers.

There are different approaches to involving all members of a family. Some therapists will meet with any member willing to attend. Unfortunately, this often means that the people who most need counseling will not be actively involved in treatment. Some therapists use their own influence to invite members to participate. Sometimes the courts will intervene and require clients with dysfunctional patterns of relating to attend family sessions. This is often seen in clients who have been involved in child abuse. As a part of reuniting families, parents may be required by court order to attend family sessions and parenting classes. Another school of thought places squarely on the family the responsibility for getting members to attend. This approach suggests that family members are masters at manipulating each other. The therapist trusts that members who desire therapy can exert an influence on those members who may be reluctant to attend. If all family members are not able to attend, the therapy does not proceed. The lack of cohesiveness is seen as an indication of the family's inability to work together and thus benefit from therapy.

Structural family therapists attempt to deal with symptoms by altering patterns of communication and relating. They work to increase awareness of and strengthen boundaries between generations. Strategic family therapists may prescribe exercises designed to affect constellations of symptoms. This may include exercises in communication, such as making "I" statements or prescribing activities. For example, a therapist might recommend that members of a family spend time alone or together in mutually satisfying activities.

Family therapy may be the most cost-effective way to deal with symptoms of dysfunction in multiple family members. For example, in theory, each child and each parent might be given their own therapist. However, this can be too costly, and issues that are a result of relationship dynamic will not be addressed.

Couples Therapy

Often, when there is distress in a relationship, it is difficult to identify a single source of the difficulty. It is said, "It takes two to tango." This is remarkably true when it comes to couples who have difficulties in relating. Since one partner may become the container of distress or symptoms, that the partner is equally involved in maladaptive patterns of relating may go unrecognized. For example, in a couple struggling with addictive issues, one partner may become involved in destructive patterns of substance abuse. At first glance, the person who is using the substances may appear to have the problem. However, investigation of the relationship will inevitably show that the nonusing partner has an investment in maintaining maladaptive patterns. Perhaps the addict's difficulty serves the function of elevating the nonusing partner to a superior status, and shifts power within the relationship to that spouse. Indeed, when we become a couple, or marry, we agree to form a dance. This dance is generally rooted in our families of origin. We seek to complete unfinished business from our families of origin with our life partner(s). This may take the form of expecting a spouse to provide nurturance that was lacking in early, formative relationships. There may be unconscious projections or transference reactions that influence patterns of relating.

Couples work is an excellent format for increasing awareness of these family-of-origin issues, as well as freeing a couple to relate in a manner based in present reality. Rather than repeating maladaptive patterns learned in original families, a couple can develop healthier forms of communication. Nondestructive methods for expression of anxiety, anger, and disappointment can be found. Effective means of conflict resolution can be employed. Working on relationship skills can be important in developing effective parenting skills. When relationship issues are resolved, the couples are more free to respond to the needs of their children.

Couples work may be useful if a separation is being considered. Divorce is a common experience, and effective methods of coping have been developed. Divorce mediation has become a valued process for couples who are dealing with issues such as child custody and property division. In divorce mediation, the focus of the couples work is on achieving a satisfactory separation. The value of the relationship may be reiterated, and its timeliness and limitations placed in perspective. Feelings related to the divorce can be discussed in an environment that is buffered by the participation of the therapist.

Senior Citizens

Older adults comprise an increasing segment of society. Professional counselors have been slow to respond to the changing needs of an aging population. Students of psychology and psychiatry are often loath to participate in settings that address an older population. I am reminded of the first day of graduate school, when a close friend loudly protested being sent to a nursing home for his first clinical rotation. Many beginning students pictured themselves working with children. The rest of us pictured ourselves working with neurotic adults, as in a Woody Allen movie. None of us was eager for a nursing-home placement. After graduating, the best reimbursement for my services came from medicare. Automatically, my services to the elderly were seen as valuable to the government. By default, I began to see elderly clients.

For those who specialize in geriatrics, experiences working with older adults can develop into a devotion and true enjoyment and appreciation for this stage in life. Older clients have special needs. Their issues and conflicts must be placed in the context of history and culture over previous decades. Developmentally, they face special challenges. There are unique physiological changes that accompany advancing years. Sadly, it is still difficult to find a practitioner who genuinely specializes in older adults. There is a great need for geropsychologists, geropsychiatrists, and general medical doctors who specialize in geriatrics.

Older adult clients can benefit significantly from ongoing contact with a psychotherapist. At times, this service must take place in the home because of difficulty with mobility or transportation. Many older adults become isolated because it is difficult for them to get around. In addition, the longer you live, the more people you know who die. Siblings and spouses pass away. Contact with a therapist or a therapy group can help ease the pain of loneliness and isolation.

Medications should be used cautiously with older adults. Metabolism slows down, so lower doses are required. Many older adults have several doctors who may prescribe drugs that can interact and produce side effects. Many drugs that are prescribed for physical symptoms may produce side effects that mimic true psychological symptoms. When an older adult comes in for an evaluation, it is important to examine current medication regimes in order to assess for psychotropic effects. The therapist may find that removing or altering drugs and doses in collaboration with the prescribing physician will alleviate symptoms of mental distress. For example, some medications for hypertension can induce feelings of depression. Steroids may produce personality changes, irritability, and altered perceptions. Older adults are at risk for polypharmacy (too many types of medications). It is not infrequent for an elderly client to suddenly develop confusion, memory difficulty, or disorientation as a result of the interactions of medications for physical disabilities. In addition, clients who have psychological symptoms treated with pharmacological interventions need to be monitored closely. Some drugs are more appropriate for elderly clients. Medications may be prescribed in smaller doses.

The therapist who works with older adult clients must understand the special issues facing them. Later years involve making an adjustment to a fixed income. Many older adults live in poverty. Physical complaints take on increasing importance. Studies show that older adults are not so much afraid of dying as they are of becoming ill and placing a burden on care givers.

Many normal physical and mental changes accompany

growing old. Muscles lose their strength, bones become brittle and fragile, and memory and problem-solving abilities change. Appetite and sleep patterns may also change. However, there are several signs that are not normal. Depression is not normal. Confusion or memory difficulty is not normal. If an older adult experiences these symptoms, consultation with a health professional should be initiated. It is not normal to become depressed in later years. Even though there are losses and changes in life-style, feelings of sadness should be transient.

Form

Once you decide you want to get started in therapy, the issue of treatment setting becomes important. There are a number of places and physical structures where you can participate in therapy programs. The most common settings for treatment include private offices and hospitals that specialize in mental health. However, additional treatment settings and structures may be beneficial. In addition to private consultation rooms and inpatient units, there are day and evening programs, support groups, in-home services, and residential programs.

Which setting is best for you depends on your individual needs. It is important to consider the amount of support and structure that is needed in the environment. Most people can work on psychological problems through intermittent contact in a therapist's office. Knowing that the therapist is available in case of emergencies and that regular contact is scheduled provides enough support to work through even the tough issues. However, some people need more support than is offered in outpatient work. If someone needs more continuous contact with care givers—either in times of crisis or early in treatment—an inpatient setting might be more useful. If physical needs must be addressed, such as for someone elderly or someone physiologically addicted to drugs, then an inpatient setting may be the safest place to begin treatment. If a client has uncontrollable impulses to hurt himself or others, then a structured environment may be needed until he can independently manage them. Questions should be asked about how much stress the client can manage on their own and what kind of support network, including family and friends, is available.

The client's strengths and limitations in emotional and psychological functioning must be considered. Is the client able to contain emotions and talk about impulses rather than acting on them? Can the client tolerate anxiety and difficult feelings between sessions without interfering with meeting daily goals? Can the client plan and direct her own well-being without the aid of a therapist or counselor? Is reality-testing accurate and reliable?

Another factor that affects choice of treatment setting is funding. The types of services covered by insurance and third-party payors frequently influence where treatment will be obtained. For example, ten years ago insurance policies were relatively generous in paying for inpatient hospitalization. Clients with chronic mental illness would often come to the hospital for several weeks in order to manage difficult symptoms. Funding for treatment outside the hospital was limited, and frequently the client would be discharged to the care of her family, without professional follow-up. Today, the tables have turned. Coverage for inpatient treatment has been dramatically reduced, so hospital stays are short. Reimbursement for day treatment and partial hospitalization is more generous. Much of the care that was previously provided in hospitals for these clients is now provided in day programs and partial hospital programs. There are pros and cons to each system of delivery of care. In the old days, some people were kept in institutions much too long simply because it was paid for. Some clients who might have been able to live in the community were not allowed access to outpatient or day-treatment programs because financial support for these options was not available. On the other hand, today, some people who might benefit from extended hospitalization or extensive treatment support are being managed as outpatients and fending for themselves in the community because financial resources for inpatient programs have dried up.

In addition to financial resources, treatment setting depends on the resources available in the client's environment. Places of employment frequently can offer support. There may be local self-help groups that can supplement professional interventions. The types of clinical resources in the community may also influence choices of settings.

A client has the legal right to receive treatment in the least-restrictive environment. This means that if outpatient treatment is sufficient, inpatient treatment cannot be substituted against the client's will. If a client will participate voluntarily in treatment, involuntary commitment cannot be used instead. (This will be discussed in greater depth later in the chapter.)

Outpatient Treatment

Outpatient treatment is available in private offices and community mental health centers. Many hospitals have therapists who provide services in an outpatient department. Outpatient psychotherapy is best suited to clients who are able to cope successfully with the demands of daily living. Relatively speaking, the client best suited to outpatient therapy is able to work and maintain relationships that support adapting to life's daily stresses. Life may present challenges, but the client best suited to outpatient work is able to effectively solve most problems, in most situations. Outpatient treatment can be used if a client is able to refrain from acting on impulses to harm themselves or others.

The client must be capable of working in sessions, then using the information between sessions. If any disturbing emotions arise in session, the client can be aware of them and hold them in mind, to be worked on in the next session. While an increasing awareness of emotions and psychological patterns may be somewhat unpleasant or disturbing, it does not destabilize the person's personality or overwhelm their coping resources. Daily life continues despite working through any upsetting psychological issues. The outpatient client, in general, will have a realistic perception of reality and is not troubled by hallucinations, confusion, or delusions.

Inpatient Treatment

The decision to voluntarily enter the hospital is generally shared between therapist—most often a psychiatrist—and the client. A psychiatrist becomes involved in the decision to advise hospitalization because only psychiatrists can admit patients to a hospital. (There are a few exceptions. Some states allow psychologists hospital-admission privileges.) In addition, a representative of the insurance company is generally involved in the decision to use inpatient treatment. Because costs are so high they cannot be absorbed out of pocket by most individuals.

At times, a client will become aware of an increased need for support and structure. Clients have a good sense about whether they can cope with the demands of a crisis in everyday life. I have learned to consider it seriously when a client says, "I think I need to go to the hospital." Often, when a client is describing severe symptoms, I ask, "Do *you* think you need to go to the hospital?" Clients are often able to identify when they are unable to cope alone, either because of altered perception of reality or destructive impulses that threaten to get out of control.

Clients sometimes have unrealistic ideas about going into the hospital. They say, "I need a vacation from my life," and imagine a hospital setting much like a spa or sanctuary from stress. They picture getting some rest and having nursing assistants catering to their every whim twenty-four hours a day. The days of checking into the sanitarium for a peaceful rest and quiet introspection are gone. Clients in a hospital are seriously impaired, and the focus of treatment is a self-care model. Clients in a mental health unit are expected to actively work on treatment goals.

Today, inpatient treatment is for the client who is having difficulty with impulse-control or reality-testing. It may also be appropriate to consider inpatient treatment when clients who have complex medical histories begin to take psychotropic medications. In a hospital, staff can closely monitor for effects and side effects of medications. When symptoms are so severe that a client can no longer manage activities of daily living, inpatient treatment may be most appropriate. For example, if a client with depression has such severe lethargy that they have given up bathing and eating, inpatient intervention may be necessary.

In most institutions, bed costs on an inpatient unit range from $800 to $1,200 a day. In addition, there are separate charges for physician and psychologist services and medications. Because it is so expensive, inpatient treatment should be reserved for clients with serious symptoms.

The amount of time a patient spends in the hospital may vary, depending on the success of treatment interventions. Thankfully, the process of deinstitutionalization has brought an end to lifetime hospitalization. In the past, clients with severe mental illness often became permanent residents of inpatient units. State hospital systems provided care to individuals sometimes for more than fifty years. Today, clients who need ongoing daily support are encouraged to live in residential settings where staff can provide care via community living assistance. Today, hospital stays are relatively brief. Depending on the needs of the client and the amount of treatment covered by insurance, clients tend to stay in the hospital for several days to several weeks. It is becoming increasingly frequent for some clients to spend hours in a hospital setting in order to achieve stabilization during a crisis, and then be discharged to a less restrictive setting. Naturally, there will always be a few clients whose needs exceed what is provided in a community setting. Unfortunately, with changes in the funding structure, the number of places providing ongoing hospitalization is disappearing. We have yet to find a balance of treatment settings that we are willing to fund in order to meet a majority of mental health needs.

Inpatient treatment offers a highly structured environment, with a daily schedule and clear behavioral expectations. For example, in a hospital, meals occur at regular times, and there are guidelines about how to interact with staff members and other clients. Group therapies occur with regularity, and expectations in group meetings can be made clear. This structure may be a welcome relief from the chaos that may have been characteristic of the client's life-style prior to admission.

Once a client enters a hospital, he undergoes a formal evaluation process. This generally involves interviews, observation in the milieu, and a physical exam. A treatment plan is developed with the client, and goals for the hospitalization are established. Diagnostic tests might be scheduled to rule out any biological factors contributing to symptoms. Interventions might include individual meetings with a therapist, psychiatrist, or counselor. Group meetings may be helpful in developing coping skills and garnering feedback on behavior and perceptions. The milieu, with its support and social order, may provide relief of anxiety and other symptoms.

The benefits of hospitalization include being able to support the client in a safe environment. A thorough assessment and evaluation of current difficulties can be performed. Intervention can be closely monitored for effectiveness. Clinicians are close by in order to deal with severe symptoms or side effects of medications. However, there may be side effects to hospitalization itself, since it artificially removes the client from his natural environment. Although this may provide temporary relief, the client must eventually return to the stressful situation, and thus may experience a return of symptoms. For treatment effects to be realistically evaluated, the client must be in his usual setting.

Self-perception is changed, perhaps permanently, by hospitalization. Some people can take the need for hospitalization in stride and view it without stigma. However, for others, being hospitalized may contribute to a lowered self-esteem. Society continues to harbor lingering prejudices about the need for inpatient psychiatric treatment. Using a hospital for treatment may support unhealthy wishes for dependence as well as helplessness as a coping style. This is called secondary gain, and refers to the gratification a client receives as a result of her illness and symptoms. For example, a client who feels lonely and empty most of the time might enjoy the company of others while staying in an inpatient unit. However, having staff members artificially available to quell feelings of loneliness does not encourage the client to develop social skills that can be used at home. The client who becomes too dependent on a hospital setting will have a difficult time returning to her own home.

Clients are sometimes unprepared to see the level of distress encountered in other patients in an inpatient unit. For example, if a client who comes to the hospital for depression is placed in a unit with other clients who are out of touch with reality, it may be a frightening experience. Clients with less severe symptoms may wonder, "Am I really as sick as they are?" and suffer further blows to self-esteem. Depending on the level of professional care delivered, inpatient settings are sometimes tense and frightening places. To the layperson, seeing someone being restrained for their own protection might be overwhelming and hard to understand. When restraints are used appropriately, they can help a client regain behavioral control while preventing injury. However, witnessing someone being restrained is often upsetting. With adequate staff support, clients with diverse needs can be cared for in inpatient settings.

Partial Hospitalization

A partial-hospitalization program involves day treatment for clients who have significant mental health needs. This treatment setting offers many of the benefits of inpatient treatment but allows the client to return home at the end of the day. Most partial programs include a schedule of group activities and psychotherapies. Groups can address common issues, including the need for social and emotional support, building skills, and problem solving. The focus of group content might be social skills, current events, life-skills training, and supportive or insight-oriented therapy.

Partial-hospitalization programs include opportunities for individual therapy and medication-management. As part of a comprehensive program, clients will participate in those aspects of treatment that meet individual needs. Families are encouraged to participate in some aspects of the partial-hospitalization program.

Evening treatment programs can be highly effective in helping a client maintain employment while receiving needed treatment. Substance-abuse treatment programs were quick to adopt this form of treatment in order to allow employees to receive maximal support while continuing to work during the day.

Residential Treatment

Community-living arrangements can allow clients to benefit from staff support for activities of daily living. Residential treatment is often combined with a partial-hospitalization program during the day. Clients can receive the benefits of a supported living situation and treatment in a community-based setting. This form of support for people with chronic mental illness has gained increasing popularity as deinstitutionalization programs continue to release clients from long-term hospital treatment. In this setting, staff members help clients manage the tasks of running a household, interacting socially, and getting to and from treatment programs. Staff members help with shopping, cleaning, reminding clients to take medications, and solving problems that might arise between members sharing a household. Staff members in these settings are generally available twenty-four hours a day but come and go in shifts rather than live with clients. This alternative is considered preferable to institutionalization, as the clients get the benefits of living in a community for about the same costs. There are some drawbacks, however, in that many communities are not so welcoming to group homes for clients with chronic mental illness. Ideally, these group homes were to be integrated into an accepting community. In reality, most communities have residents who are afraid of people with chronic mental illness, and there can be vehement protests from communities before accepting this type of arrangement. Once a community-living arrangement is established, often, the members are not integrated but isolated from other community members.

In-Home Services

Several forms of treatment may take place in the client's home. For example, a behavioral therapist might begin working in the home with a client who is agoraphobic. At times, the treatment of choice for children involves providing family support in the home. In addition, clients who are homebound because of illness or aging can receive psychiatric and psychological services in their own home. A house call may be just what the doctor orders! Interventions in this setting have a tendency to be highly effective, as the therapist can gain a comprehensive understanding of the client's situation by being in the very setting. A home visit is ideal for involving family members and assessing family dynamics. Home visits cannot provide social interaction, and if appropriate, in-home counseling can lead to the client's having increased mobility and participation in outpatient services. Insurance will often consider reimbursing these services, if the client is home-bound and cannot get to an office, or the home-based treatment is the most cost-effective choice because it can prevent hospitalization.

Community Mental Health Centers

During the early 1960s, President Kennedy enacted legislation to guarantee access to mental health treatment for everyone. This legislation led to the community mental health or catchment area system. The country is divided into geographic regions or catchment areas designed to provide inpatient, outpatient, vocational, and emergency mental health services for its residents. Look for the community mental health center in your local phone book. This is a public system, so waiting lists for available appointments may be long. Clinicians are often underskilled and overworked. However, many dedicated and skilled providers make a career in this system and provide admirable services. Students also use these sites as part of their training, so a talented student may be found in the local Community Mental Health Center. Treatment is provided at a minimal fee.

Integrated Delivery Systems

Serious mental health symptoms sometimes become chronic in nature. Clients with chronic mental illness generally receive treatment in a combination of settings. When symptoms are exacerbated, the client may go into the hospital for crisis-management. After being discharged from the hospital, they may be referred to a partial-hospitalization program and an individual therapist. When symptoms are in remission, maintenance outpatient therapy visits may be sufficient to monitor for increasing symptoms. Choices about treatment setting need not be an either/or proposition. Treatment may take place in several settings simultaneously to better address specific client needs.

Psychological Testing

Psychological testing is a useful tool for obtaining a rapid, detailed assessment of strengths and weaknesses in thinking and personality. Intelligence testing became popular during the early 1960s, and most school children have an intellectual evaluation as a part of elementary-school routine. Intelligence testing is done by giving the client a variety of tasks that requires them to use a wide range of skills to respond. For example, there might be items that tap into information you learned formally in school, or tasks that call upon memory or social skills. The idea is that intelligence is made up of a number of factors and ways of thinking, some of which show up in school testing and others that show up in artistic, creative, or even athletic ways. Because intelligence-test results have been misused for purposes of political discrimination, protections have been enacted so that labels are applied cautiously and judiciously. Conclusions about intelligence are never reached on the basis of a single instrument. In addition, behavioral observations of the person must look at his real-life abilities. Some of the common instruments that are used with children include the Weschler Intelligence Scale for Children; the Stanford Binet; or the Writing, Reading, Arithmetic Test. School psychologists employ a battery of instruments to best assess a child's abilities and design programs to remediate areas of difficulty to achieve the greatest academic success. In adults, intellectual functioning can be assessed with the Weschler Adult Intelligence Scales. These tests sample a wider range of cognitive abilities and can screen for areas of difficulty, as well as areas of ability.

In addition to intellectual assessment, psychologists can offer a wide range of vocational testing. A number of assessment tools can be used to assess aptitudes and interests. There are tools that can assess work-skill strengths and communication patterns and styles. The Myers Briggs evaluation tool has been widely used in work settings to assess different styles of relating and working together. When a work group takes the Myers Briggs inventory together, they can compare styles of interacting, and then design work patterns that utilize individual employee's strengths within a team.

Measuring and evaluating personality and emotional functioning is a blend of art and science. Personality is assessed through tests that look at patterns of thinking and emotion. These are inventories that survey preferences to determine personality style, such as the Minnesota Multiphasic Personality Inventory. There are surveys about symptoms such as the Millon Clinical Multiaxial Inventory, or the Symptoms Checklist (SCLR-90).

In addition to the quantitative self-report measures, psychologists use projective testing to assess personality. A projective test involves the use of the client's mental activities to come up with a response to an item. For example, if an item asks, "How much is two plus two?" it pulls for a structured, arithmetic response that does not necessarily involve the use of personality style or emotions. The most common answer would undoubtedly be four. If a client replies "five" or "I hate math" to the question, he is using some personality and emotion to render an answer. Projective tests have varying degrees of structure.

In the Thematic Apperception Test, a client is shown real-life pictures and asked to make up a story with a beginning, middle, and an end. The client makes up the stories using his personality, but the pictures are of real objects.

Another projective test involves drawing pictures. The client is instructed to draw a person, a tree, or a house. This is somewhat structured, because trees, people, and houses bring some idea to mind, but to draw them on a blank page involves using our personality and emotional style. In the Rorschach inkblot test, the client is shown random patterns of ink, with no actual structure, and asked, "What might this look like?" The stimulus has little structure, requiring the client to use a great deal of her personality to produce a response.

In the early years of personality assessment, ideas were generated from the clinician's educated impressions. For example, the client was shown an inkblot and asked what it might look like. He replies, "a birthday cake." If there was more evidence supporting this in the rest of the tests, the evaluating clinician might conclude that he is a happy person who enjoys celebrations. Today, assessment of inkblot responses is much more scientific. We have collected data on millions of clients internationally, with all manner of personality functioning. We have collected statistical norms that tell us how often a client will see a birthday cake, and what types of people are most likely to see birthday cakes. We have also developed several objective ways to score responses to ambiguous tests such as those to quantify our results and conclusions. However, part of the art of personality-test interpretation remains, as the clinician compares his objective results with subjective impressions during the testing and makes an assessment of personality and emotional functioning. A clinician must do hundreds of these in order to become an expert and to calibrate himself into an accurate assessment instrument capable of integrating scientific and intuitive data.

Psychological testing is often used in situations where

there is a legal question, such as custody evaluation or in criminal cases. Forensic psychologists and psychiatrists have developed a unique subspecialty and specific instruments that are added to a standard battery for assessment purposes. Psychological testing tends to be costly and frequently is not covered by insurance companies. If testing is needed but you cannot afford it, it may be available at a reduced cost through local universities with graduate psychology programs. In custody or criminal cases, testing may be done by court-appointed providers. However, if you are planning to support a legal case you are building with expert psychological testimony and testing, these costs will be out of pocket. Most lawyers who do this type of work have a number of forensic psychologists and psychiatrists with whom they collaborate routinely.

Content

Theoretical Approaches

In addition to the various structures and forms of therapy that may be implemented, different theoretical approaches to treatment must be considered. You may be wondering which type of therapy would be best for you. There are behavioral approaches, cognitive approaches, and dynamic approaches. How to begin and which one is best for you is an important issue and should be discussed and considered carefully. As mentioned in chapter 1, it is important to match the treatment, client, and situation individually.

The matching process occurs as you interview and consult various prospective therapists. You may wish to share a brief summary of the problem with the therapist and ask what treatment they would recommend. A therapist might recommend an active collaboration or a more extensive evaluation.

You can ask the therapist outright what theoretical approach they use, but unless you are well acquainted with the available options, the answer might be less than meaningful.

Clients self-select treatment approaches. A client will search for a therapist who can offer interventions that are in keeping with her own personality style. For example, a client who is uncomfortable with dependency might feel best in an active collaboration that involves behavioral exercises. A client who is naturally introspective might feel most at home with dynamic therapy. If the treatment offered doesn't match the client's preferred mode of operating, the client generally moves on. Clients also evaluate the type of support offered by a therapist. Interpersonal warmth is a critical factor for some clients, while others look for intellectual attributes.

If a client unknowingly begins to work with a therapist who offers an approach that does not match his understanding, he may use the new method for a time. If it is helpful, it may be incorporated, and the therapy will continue. If the method is of limited benefit, the client generally breaks off treatment, perhaps using the therapist's perspective to change an aspect of the presenting problem.

It is important that you realize there are many methods of working in therapy. It is not unusual to have to interview several therapists before you find a good fit. Do not be discouraged. Many therapists are capable of implementing treatments from a broad range of approaches, and adaptations can be made as a plan of approach is developed. If you want a treatment approach that the therapist does not offer, for example, medications or hypnosis, the therapist may refer you to a colleague or collaborate with another therapist.

Every theory contributes to our understanding. At different times in working through issues, we may need a variety of perspectives to reach our goals. For example, a client with relationship difficulties consulted with a psychoanalyst and a social work counselor at different times during his development.

The psychoanalyst encouraged understanding the unconscious aspects of the relationship difficulties, which was accomplished with good results. The social worker suggested that relationships needed to be experienced, and encouraged interacting in social settings. The client did this also, with good results. Different perspectives need not compete and can be implemented serially or simultaneously.

Each therapist utilizes an array of scientific theories to develop an effective, individualized treatment approach. Clinicians and clients bring with them to the work ideas about psychosocial functioning. These unique perspectives will have a powerful impact on the way issues are approached in-session. For example, if a client has a strong belief that early childhood experiences have a strong influence on current experiences, and a therapist believes that a combination of the past and present contributes to current adaptation, these participants may evolve a therapy that looks at early childhood functioning and current difficulties. The theories that guide exploration come from both the client and the therapist. A good-enough therapist uses a wide variety of theories to tailor the therapy to the client's individual perspectives.

Rights and Responsibilities in Treatment: Confidentiality and Privilege

Privilege is the client's legal right stemming from privacy laws. The laws of privacy dictate that the client has a right to decide who has access to confidential information. You control the release of information about yourself. The therapist cannot reveal information discussed in-session unless the client gives explicit written permission about what information may be revealed and to whom.

Confidentiality is the therapist's legal duty; it stems from anti-gossip laws. The therapist has a duty not to reveal information unless the client's consent has been obtained. This duty prevents the therapist from talking or writing about sessions to others. If a client is involved in research or the therapist is interested in writing about some aspect of the contact, the client must consent to this in writing, and the therapist must make every effort to disguise or protect the client's identity.

There are some exceptions to privilege and confidentiality. The legal and clinical professions have collectively made a judgment that in some situations, the good of society as a whole or the need to protect individuals may supersede the need for privacy. A therapist is wise to discuss these exceptions to confidentiality and privilege at the outset of a therapy in order to avoid confusion or misunderstanding at a later date. This presents an interesting dilemma. The therapist should explain that she will report to appropriate authorities a client's intentions to commit certain acts of violence. If the client tells the therapist, she will respond accordingly in order to prevent any violence. The client will realize that if he doesn't want the therapist to intervene, he must not reveal any intentions to harm himself or others. If the therapist advises the client of the limits of confidentiality, she runs the risk that the client will not reveal these thoughts in-session. For example, therapists are mandated by law to report to appropriate channels a situation that may involve the abuse of a child, dependent, or elder. If during the course of psychotherapy, a therapist has reason to suspect that the client is abusing a child, or if the client is a child and is being abused, she is legally bound to alert child welfare authorities of her suspicions and to alert them to the need for an investigation.

If a therapist believes that a client is in imminent danger of harming himself, the therapist has the authority to act on the client's behalf to protect him from harm. This may involve alerting family members of the wish to self-harm or to initiate an involuntary commitment process. If the therapist has reason to believe that the client is in danger of harming someone else, she has a duty to warn others of the danger. This may involve but not be limited to alerting family, law enforcement, the intended victim, and/or initiating an involuntary commitment. The legal precedent for these situations stems from the Tarasoff decision in California, in which a therapist was seeing a young man who talked of harming a female coed at a local university. The therapist did alert local authorities and attempted to initiate an involuntary commitment. However, before preventive action could be taken, the client murdered the coed. The client's family successfully sued the therapist, saying he should have warned the intended victim and her family. Since that decision, the actions of a therapist treating a client who may harm another have not been limited to prescribed actions; instead, the therapist must do whatever is necessary to protect the potential victim. These laws apply only to violent acts that the client may be contemplating. They do not involve reporting previous violent acts. Thus, a client who reveals that he has murdered someone in the past is protected from having the therapist reveal that information to use against him much in the same way that a defense attorney is prevented from revealing his client's guilt.

Additional exceptions to confidentiality involve court orders. A court can order a therapist to reveal certain information such as a divorce in legal proceedings. If a therapist is ordered by a court to testify about information revealed in therapy sessions, she is ethically and legally mandated to reveal information specific to the question at hand, and only information that is relevant. Most therapists will refuse to turn over notes or transcripts of sessions, preferring to testify in person about pertinent questions. Clients should also be aware that if they bring a legal action where their therapy or mental health is a central issue, privilege will be waived. For example, if someone sues for mental suffering after a motor vehicle accident, records from therapy will not be protected in a court of law. Likewise, if a client sues a therapist for malpractice, records from the treatment will no longer be considered privileged.

Given existing requirements for reimbursement from managed-care companies, there is a growing concern about the ability to protect confidentiality. Many insurance companies require detailed information about the nature of symptoms and treatment before they will authorize payment for services. Therapists are under an obligation to report only information that is relevant to the reimbursement process. Clients have a right to know and control what information is being released. Part of the problem stems from the fact that insurance companies are not necessarily bound by the same obligations to protect confidentiality as are therapists. Even when required to abide by company policies to protect the release of information, employees often have limited training and are not bound by the same ethics as a licensed professional. When information is recorded in computers or in areas where many people have access to files, the risk of information being leaked improperly becomes a grave concern. These reporting requirements are seen by some therapists as threatening the very privacy that is a necessary requirement for therapy to take place. Some clients may avoid coming to treatment because they are afraid their personal secrets will become known. Wealthier clients may be able to avoid this problem by paying for treatment out of pocket and not using their insurance benefits. There is a risk that therapy will become a privilege of the upper class and be unavailable to those who rely on third-party reimbursement for care.

Therapists who work with insurance companies walk a fine line to protect client confidentiality and to disclose enough information so that the third-party payor can determine the need for and effectiveness of treatment. For example, with the client's permission a therapist might tell the insurance company that a client has symptoms of depression, including vegetative signs that have been present for several months. Treatment might be described in terms of interventions such as assessment of symptoms, consideration of medications, and identifying behavioral goals. The therapist can communicate about progress without revealing personal details or secrets. However, we must investigate how to protect confidentiality when therapists communicate with third-party payers.

Informed Consent

Informed consent involves two elements: one of information (informed), and one of agreement (consent). It is the therapist's duty to inform the client of the risks and benefits of any intervention or treatment. The therapist has an obligation to discuss, in language that the client can understand, the structure, purpose, and goals of psychotherapy, as well as any risks of harm or side effects that may occur. The client must decide freely, without undue influence, to participate in the treatment. You should never be pressured or coerced into treatment. Protecting the client's right to choose or refuse treatment options is an obligation of the therapist, as clients who come to therapists in distress are vulnerable to promises of relief and might be easily exploited. Even clients who are committed for involuntary evaluation have rights to refuse treatment in nonemergency situations.

Informed consent should take place at the outset of treatment, and ideally, consent to treatment should be in writing. Many therapists who see private clients do not obtain a written consent because as a legal precedent, showing up voluntarily for an appointment implies consent to treatment.

Boundaries

Boundaries in therapy are necessary to establish an environment of psychological and emotional safety. Keeping appointment times to the minute helps to establish that the therapist is reliably available to the client. Boundaries involve time and place. Therapist and client meet at mutually arranged times and in specific places. When a client is consistently early or late for appointments, something is being communicated.

Boundaries also include rights to privacy and self-expression. For example, a physical boundary might be a closed door. We each need a space that can be ours alone, where we can be alone with ourselves. We need to control entry into these private spaces and say how they will be shared and with whom.

A boundary refers to the dividing line between self and others. Physically, boundaries may be clear and easily observed. It is common sense to know where your body ends and where another's begins. If someone violates a physical boundary, such as in an assault, it is easy to identify where injury has occurred. Psychologically, boundaries may be more difficult to discern. In relationships, we allow the psyche of others to influence our own mental functioning. There may be some shared mind space. Because of unconscious processes, such as projection, it is sometimes difficult to tell where one person's psyche ends and another's begins.

Respect for the integrity of the therapy relationship demands that physical safety be unquestionable. The client and therapist have the right not to be touched in treatment. This means that whether it is in anger or in sensuality, physical contact will not occur. Impulses must be discussed, not acted upon. If the client is fearful that talking about fantasies and impulses might lead to behavioral expression, exploration of these aspects of mental functioning will be less likely to occur. When the client is assured that sexual impulses will never be acted upon, they are free to examine with the therapist thoughts and feelings related to sexuality.

Contact that occurs outside the office can have a powerful impact on the relationship. For the client, learning about the therapist's personal life might be overstimulating. There is a natural curiosity that evolves out of having limited information. Seeing the therapist's car, for instance, adds information to the client's ideas about the therapist. Make, model, and year tell you something about identity, interests, and socioeconomic status. Seeing each other in a public setting, such as a shopping mall, will, in part, feel like a boundary violation. The therapist inadvertently appears in the client's real world. This is an intrusion, partially welcomed, partially feared.

Least-Restrictive Alternative

Clients have the right to receive treatment in a manner that provides the fewest amount of restrictions to constitutional freedom. For example, if a client can safely be maintained in an unlocked unit, he cannot be held in a locked unit against his wishes. If a client is able to maintain appropriate behavior, seclusion and restraints will not be used. The levels of restriction involve limiting a client's movements and autonomous functioning. The least-restrictive treatment is voluntary outpatient therapy. Voluntary hospitalization involves an agreement to remain in an institution but allows freedom of movement on the grounds. Involuntary hospitalization is reserved for clients who present a danger to themselves or others, and who do not recognize the need for treatment. Movements may be restricted to a locked unit, but the client can walk around that unit unrestrained.

If a client is unable to keep himself from acting on harmful impulses, restraints of behavior may be necessary. The least-restrictive restraint is chemical, or the administration pharmacotherapy. Antipsychotic drugs may allow a client to control behavior so that free ambulation is possible. If physical restraints become necessary, great precautions must be taken to use them only as long as necessary. Locked seclusion may assist a client to regain control, while separating him from other clients. If seclusion alone is not helpful, a client may be restrained at the wrists and ankles until behavioral control is achieved. If a client needs to be restrained, a staff member should be at arm's length at all times to monitor safety and offer emotional support. Restraints are used to assist a client to regain behavioral control and prevent them from inflicting harm on self or others. Restraints are never to be used as a punishment.

Right to Treatment

Unfortunately, in this society, there is no legally established precedent that creates a right to have treatment. However, protection for *access* to treatment was established by the Johnson/Kennedy Administration. During this administration, the community mental health system was established, guaranteeing that every citizen shall have access to local facilities offering inpatient and outpatient treatment and emergency services. This later was expanded to include access to partial-hospitalization programs and vocational training. However, in general, payment for these services remains the client's responsibility unless certain standards of poverty are met. In our current legislative environment, mental health treatment is a privilege, not a right.

Right to Terminate Treatment

You have a right to stop treatment at anytime. The client has a right to terminate treatment whenever she wishes, unless a court has mandated treatment. The client has a right to decide to seek a second opinion or a consultation about therapy with another therapist at anytime. Therapists have an obligation not to abandon clients and to make referrals upon request and when clinically indicated. Therapists should cooperate in facilitating consultation.

Right to Refuse Treatment

A client does, however, have the right to refuse treatment, even if he is incarcerated or involuntarily committed. This right stems from a constitutional protection of self-determination. As a society we believe that only the client should make decision about his own body. Only a court can remove the right to refuse treatment, and most decisions protect this right in all but the most dire circumstances.

CHAPTER 6

Psychodynamic Therapy

P sychodynamic therapy is an opporunity for knowing your inner self. It differs from other forms of psycho-therapy because it focuses on hidden forces in the mind and encourages the client to use insight and understanding as a method of resolution of difficulties. The therapist is support-ive but nondirective, acting as a faciltator on the journey. Un-less there is a specific reason to be directive, the therapist's role in dynamic therapy is to offer insight and observation in a way that allows the client to discover his own true self, and true path. Dynamic therapy looks at how previous events in life, particularly early life experiences, can contribute to the shape of things today. Other therapies, such as behavioral or cognitive approaches (discussed in the next chapter), focus on more obvious aspects of functioning, such as action or thought. The therapist is relatively more active and directive. The focus is on the here and now rather than on previous events.

Beginning to understand the hidden forces of the mind, you can come to understand how mental or psychic events de-termine what goes on in your life. Initially, some people are skeptical that an unconscious exists. However, when you begin to be aware of the evidence of unconscious activity, it is hard to disregard these profound phenomena. Evidence that there are unconscious forces at work include repetitive patterns of behavior, dreams, slips of the tongue, and symptoms.

Dynamic therapy works with the structure of the mind. Ideally, your personality and psychological abilities function in a way that allows you to easily meet the demands of everyday reality. The ego balances the demands of the id and the admonitions of the superego. Growing up, we need experiences that allow us to develop a strong sense of self, an accurate understanding of reality, the ability to think effectively, and to experience fully a wide range of emotions. Dynamic therapy works with the aftereffects of life experiences that have been traumatic or inadequate in providing essential elements for growth. For example, if there were many secrets in your family of origin, therapy can provide an opportunity for experiencing a relationship that is rooted in honesty. As you discuss subjects that were taboo in your family, the therapeutic process helps to reduce shame. Or if you are struggling with a sense of inadequacy, dynamic therapy can uncover the roots of these feelings and help you build a healthier sense of self.

Symptoms are understood as coming from conflicting forces within the mind or limitations in the dynamic functioning of the mind. A conflict is basically a situation of wanting two things at the same time. If you are sitting reading this book but at the same time wishing you could get up and go for a walk, then you are experiencing a conflict. This is a minor conflict, easily resolved by either continuing to read, or taking a walk, and coming back later to finish reading.

Dynamic therapy views people within the context of relationships. Who we are is understood as being embedded in reciprocal interactions and interdependence. Who and how we are is, in part, due to the relationships we participate in. In addition to studying relationships in general, dynamic therapy uses the therapist-client relationship as a mechanism for change. The relationship with the therapist can be studied closely, partly because of the therapist's self-awareness. Unconscious patterns that are superimposed on most relationships also express themselves within the therapy relationship. When these distortions are illuminated, they can be worked through and eliminated, allowing current relationships to exist more freely.

Psychodynamic therapy places a unique value on subjective experience, and the therapist attempts to see the world as the client sees it. The clients perceptions of reality are what need to be worked with, because this information determines how the person thinks and acts. The goal of the adult client is to perceive accurately reality and be able to respond to it in an effective, mature way with a wide range of choices. Together the client and therapist look for distortions in how things really are. When distortions are found, they can be examined for validity.

For example, a client might begin to notice that in situations that would make most people angry, she does not express anger. She and the therapist begin to note the absence of appropriate anger and wonder how this came to be. In thinking back on early family experiences, they discover a family standard of never expressing anger directly. It was viewed as morally incorrect, and messages to the children were clear, "You are not to feel, or talk about, or even have angry feelings." As an adult, this client carried forward this guideline for behavior learned in her early family. When the rule was discovered, it was examined for validity. The client found herself developing ulcers and migraines. At times, coworkers would take advantage of her because of her fear of expressing any hint of anger. The reality of life is that we all feel angry at times; it is a natural human emotion and should be accepted and validated when appropriate. With the recognition of this unconscious rule, and a conscious choice to experiment with it, the client began to make changes in how she handled angry feelings. She told the therapist about things that made her angry. Slowly, she began to confront her coworkerss. Gradually, the client realized that she was not a bad person because she experienced feelings of anger. When she shared her angry feelings with the therapist, she took a huge risk and broke the no-talk rule. Her shame decreased and her self-acceptance improved. Her identity became stronger as the thereapist validated these feelings rather than perpetuating denial and distortion.

While Freud is credited with being first to realize that talking through emotional difficulties can bring relief, he actually worked with a number of people to develop his ideas. Freud was a young physician struggling to make a living and a name for himself in Vienna in the 1880s. He began working with Joseph Breurer to treat patients with neurological disorders. He was working with techniques developed in France by Jean Charcot and began using hypnosis to produce improvement in neurological symptoms. He discovered that when his patients underwent hypnosis and talked about the symptoms during this highly relaxed state, they improved. Freud theorized that this might, in part, be because symptoms had a psychological basis that sustained them rather than a purely physical basis. For example, a man with a paralyzed arm but with no obvious psysiological cause would undergo hypnosis, talk about when the symptoms began, and then upon awakening, would find his arm fully functioning. In a state of hypnosis, the patient might recall the symptoms began at the same time he was having a thought about using his arm in a violent way, or more often in some socially unacceptable sexual way. It was as if his mind had paralyzed his arm in order to inhibit these unacceptable impulses and protect him from the consequences of acting on them. Freud wondered at the power of what he called *unconscious* forces of the mind being able to produce such dramatic symptoms.

Although the hypnotic state was helpful in reducing symptoms, at times, upon awakening, patients would forget what they had discovered about the psychological aspects of the symptoms, and the value of the treatment was lost. Freud began to experiment with techniques that involved talking about symptoms, without the hypnotic trance, and the talking cure was born.

Psychodynamic therapy is the modern version of the talking cure. Although Freud is credited with being the first to develop psychoanalytic theory, is has been contributed to for almost 100 years, and includes the work of many talented clinicians. Several fundamental beliefs comprise the theory of dynamic treatment. The first is the relative importance of unconscious processes. Dynamic therapists believe that unconscious forces have a powerful impact on feelings and actions. Although we believe we are consciously in control of our behavior, in reality, our unconscious mental activities largely determine our experience. Dynamic therapy assumes that there are no psychological accidents. Theory suggests that mental activity, behaviors, and feelings all make sense when they are understood in the context of the conscious and unconscious forces of the mind. In other words, actions and symptoms are not random, they have meaning. This is called psychic determinism, which assumes that there is continuity in mental life, and that what occurs unconsciously is directly related to what happens consciously. For example, even when a dream appears to come out of nowhere, it can actually be traced back to understandable mental events. In addition, dynamic therapists believe that "the child is father to the man," and that previous experiences have a profound impact on the present.

The process of dynamic therapy involves suspending

some of our logical, goal-oriented, realistic thinking (as can happen artifically with hypnosis), and talking about whatever comes to mind in regard to symptoms, conflicts, thoughts, and feelings. Talking through concerns allows the therapist and patient to observe mental life; thus, the client develops a dynamic understanding of herself. With an understanding of mental forces that are in operation, you can have more conscious choice about how you react and behave in life. Through therapy we may become less fearful about our inner mental life, and as a result we are more accepting of who we are and less judgmental about human experience. We can become more able to participate fully in life's experiences rather than using our energy to protect ourselves from danger, criticism, and emotional injury.

Psychoanalytic psychotherapy uses the method of free association to observe conscious and unconscious functioning. The client and the analyst takes a position of observation that is equidistant from the id, ego, and superego. In other words, traces of functioning from each of these three areas of the mind should be regarded with equal respect. A balanced observation attempts to foster an environment that does not promote censorship of any mental activities.

Lester Luborsky, a noted researcher at the University of Pennsylvania, characterized treatment as having supportive and expressive aspects. Supportive interactions involve positive reinforcement of the client's self or ego functions. example, a therapist may support decisions made during problem solving and note the client's strengths in functioning. Expressive aspects of therapy include talking about issues, feelings, and conflicts. Expressive elements involve catharsis, or the release of emotion.

Although Freud analyzed himself (the only person to successfully use this solitary method), psychodynamic therapy or analysis is by nature a relationship. It is a unique relationship because it is circumscribed by specific boundaries of time and place. It is available for study, like no other ordinary relationship. The analyst, as a part of her training, develops a deep knowledge of herself and thus can avoid imposing her own conflicts onto the therapy relationship. The relationship allows both client and therapist to monitor for distortions in the relationship. They can be alert for ideas or roles that are imposed on an artificially neutral canvas. For example, if the analyst assumes a neutral position in the therapy, but the client has a history of conflict with authority figures, the client may impose an authoritarian role on the therapist and react to him as if he is an authority and not a neutral party. The client learns how these distortions, once observed, may be affecting other relationships in his life.

In addition, the therapist is also a real presence. Therapists are interested and offer sustained, consistent, predictable attention for significant episodes of time, several times a week. Having someone skillfully attend to you in this way may be different from other relationships. In addition, the therapist is supportive and nonjudgmental. The therapist is able to validate feelings and experiences. It can be a powerful transformation when you meet someone who cay say, "I understand things *just* the way you do." This validation is enormously satisfying and can result in increased self-esteem. The client borrows the therapist's positive regard for her, until she can incorporate it as positive self-regard. Over time, the therapy may provide a corrective emotional experience, offering a relationship with a real person who is accepting of the client as she actually is rather than expecting some false self to meet some role expectation. Experiencing empathy and unconditional positive regard allows the character to develop to its highest potential. We need this mirroring from somewhere in order to grow fully and mature.

Most people begin dynamic therapy with some apprehension about aspects of themselves they are afraid to face. Often, clients believe that if they don't acknowledge an issue, it won't be active—the let sleeping dogs lie approach. The opposite is generally the case. If a conflict is not acknowledged, forces that are avoided can have a profound influence on functioning. When forces of the mind are examined in the light of day, they can be brought under conscious control of choice. For example, rather than blindly reacting with rage, one can stop and think, "How do I want to react to these feelings of anger?" As you examine secret feelings and aspects of yourself that create feelings of guilt, shame decreases. For example, many people harbor guilt about aggression or anger. Our inner toddler who expresses rage through destructive tantrums lurks near the surface, threatening to emerge when we experience frustration or stress. If as adults we have allowed the inner toddler behavioral expression in our adult life we may feel guilty about the destructive consequences. If we stifle these impulses completely, we may develop ulcers.

Exploring for evidence of hidden aggressive feelings happens through observing the thoughts that appear in the mind. When manifestations of hidden anger are discovered, they can be addressed with the conscious mind, the adapting ego. For example, a dream may contain a symbol of anger, such as a fire, or a violent act. During waking hours, the dreamer may be unaware of angry feelings, in part, because they are unacceptable to the superego. Through understanding the symbols in the dream, the client may recognize mixed feelings about the subject of the dream. These unconscious conflicts can be more easily addressed when they are brought into consciousness, which frees the mind from all the activities involved with defending against these unacceptable impulses. More energy becomes available.

Difficulties that are conflict-based may be best suited to individual dynamic treatment. Clients with characteristic maladaptive uses of defenses may benefit from an exploratory approach. When anxieties are caused by unconscious forces and hidden conflicts, psychodynamic therapy may be most helpful in resolving difficulties.

Differences Between Counseling and Psychotherapy

It is imporatnt to understand the differences between counseling and psychotherapy. Counseling involves support and advice. Psychotherapy is a process of exploring your dynamic psychological activities and understanding your mental life within the context of psychological forces. Counseling looks at apparent, readily observable aspects of a situation. Psychotherapy deals with both the overt and the covert. Both forms of therapy provide support. Both forms of therapy may be helpful. The goals of counseling are more limited. Psychotheraphy works toward lasting personality change and ultimately self-actualization.

Counseling is generally done by somone who is a paraprofessional. In some cases, people who provide counseling have little formal training, such as in a women's shelter or a hot line. At times, counselors receive some education and supervised practice, such as an addictions or residential counselor.

Differences Between Psychoanalysis and Psychotherapy

Psychotherapy occurs in face-to-face meetings. The therapist and client sit across from each other, which allows for observation of nonverbal feedback. Meetings take place at least once a week. Psychoanalysis may involve reclining on a couch, which allows the client to more fully relax and focus. The analyst sits out of view so as not to distort the free association with nonverbal behaviors. Silences on the part of the analyst allow for maximal projection from the client. Thus, psychoanalysis offers the client less support and less mental structure than therapy. It requires that the client use his own resources rather than borrowing from the therapist's ego.

Both forms of treatment have the same aim, goals, and roughly the same process. The aim of treatment is to make the unconscious conscious, bringing it under control of the ego. Through the process of free association, or saying whatever comes to mind, the client and the therapist observe mental functioning. Together they look for evidence of unconscious functioning as a way of better knowing the self. Dreams, slips of the tongue, and humor can all be understood from the perspective of the forces of the mind that shape them.

Who Should Participate in Psychodynamic Therapy?

Years ago, there was a popular belief that psychodynamic psychotherapy was best suited for a YARVIS, or a client who was: Young, Articulate, Rich, Verbal, Intelligent, and Single. We now know that this is not necessarily true. A young client was once thought to be preferable because of the number of years needed to accomplish therapeutic goals. However, now we know that therapy can be helpful for a client of any age, from toddlers to elders. Senior citizens can achieve significant benefit from dynamic psychotherapy as a method of understanding the life they have lived and of resolving old emotional conflicts. The ability to articulate is helpful but not a necessary prerequisite for dynamic treatment. Being able to talk about feelings and thoughts facilitates free association. However, clients who are too young to have well-developed vocabulary skills can resolve conflicts through nonverbal means, such as play. Adult clients may prefer to work on issues nonverbally through artistic expression.

Rich clients were thought to be most able to afford ongoing treatment, but in most areas, dynamic therapy can be arranged at a low or minimal fee.

An average level of intelligence may be necessary to facilitate the process of introspection and understanding psychological functioning through self-observation. However, clients with below-average intellectual capacities may benefit from the supportive aspects of a psychodynamic treatment.

The idea that single clients are most suited to psychodynamic therapy stems from a belief that attachment to the therapist requires a significant amount of psychic energy. A client distracted by family and love relationships may be less engaged in the process of psychotherapy. However, it is also helpful for a client in therapy to have significant relationships other than the therapist in order to provide support and social interaction.

So you can see that the old stereotypes about who should be in dynamic therapy have changed in recent years.

Dynamic psychotherapy may be the treatment of choice when issues are related to inner conflicts or unconscious desires or emotions. Dynamic therapy is, in part, a process of making the unconscious conscious and to increase awareness of personal functioning. With increased awareness come increased choice and control of life's options. A client in dynamic psychotherapy must have relatively healthy personality and cognitive functioning. That is to say, the client must have a basic capacity for self-observation, an ability to tolerate feelings and memories that may be joyous or upsetting. They must have the capacity to sustain a working relationship with the therapist. When a comprehensive dynamic treatment is undertaken, the client must be capable of exploring sometimes unsettling aspects of unconscious functioning. The client must be able to suspend logical thought and explore associations to fantasies that may seem unacceptable at first glance.

When a client begins an hour, they relax some of their logical, adult psychological functioning and begin to play in the associations of the unconscious. This ego function is known as ARISE, which stands for the Ability to Regress in Service of the Ego. Regressing to a more playful mode allows the client to more freely explore mental forces and ideas. The client must also be able to reverse this process and suppress awareness of these illogical experiences at the end of the hour. The client needs to be able to reorganize quickly to leave the session and to attend to the everday business of life until the next session arrives. Having the ability to be flexible in perspectives and freely shift into modes of observation and free association can allow a client to participate fully in the therapy process.

Again, clients in dynamic therapy must have a capacity for self-observation. They must be able to separate some part of their consciousness that can be aware of and monitor emotions and actions. You can develop the ability to split awareness into observation and participation. This skill can be practiced. If a client doesn't have this ability, the therapy will be more supportive in nature.

The client must have the ability to sustain an interpersonal relationship with the therapist. Interpersonal skills must be sufficient to support ongoing interactions. For example, some clients who have what is called a schizoid personality are uninterested in relating with the therapist. These people rarely come to therapy voluntarily. The experience of this therapy relationship will probably be boring to both the therapist and the client. These people are distant and reluctant to disclose personal information. There is no desire to interact in a cooperative, collaborative manner.

There are other types of people who may have difficulty sustaining a relationship in therapy. Clients who have difficulty developing a positive image of their therapist, which can be internalized, may not stay in treatment. If the client sees the therapist as threatening, or intimacy as dangerous, the negative transference may overwhelm the work. To sustain the relationship the client must have the capacity for object constancy. In other words, the client needs to be able to develop an image of the therapist in her mind which she can rely on between sessions. The ability to see someone as being related to you and important in your world even when they are not physically present, is called object constancy. For example, you may not be living with your mother, but ideas and memories about her sustain a relationship even without the physical closeness. The client must be able to do this with the therapist in order to facilitate the continuity of the work. Although a client and therapist meet for only minutes during the week, the work of the therapy continues outside of sessions, in part, because of the internalized representation of the therapist. Clients often say, "I thought of what you would have said," when recounting dilemmas from between sessions.

Clients with impulse difficulty may be unable to maintain the behavioral standards necessary for ongoing psychotherapy. Many impulses arise during the course of therapy. When we feel anxious, we might wish to get up and leave a session rather than continue to sit and talk about the issues. Or we might have the impulse to act destructively. Clients in an uncovering, exploratory therapy need to be able to feel the emotions without acting them out. For example, clients with a borderline personality organization have a tendency to behave impulsively, sometimes in ways that are dangerous to themselves or others. A client who has difficulty with impulse control needs therapy that is primarily supportive.

The client must be able to respect and maintain boundaries. Contact takes place at limited times. Emergencies need to be contained within the time frame of scheduled sessions. Extra-session contact, such as phone calls, may burden the relationship and create a stress on forward progress. The client needs to be able to form a close relationship without dissolving his own sense of self or boundaries. Tolerating the dependence that develops in psychotherapy is a challenge that allows the capacity for intimacy to grow. However, many people are fearful of such closeness and interdependence because past relationships that became close or intimate have had damaging consequences. This is particularly true for clients who have been abused or abandoned in early experiences.

The Method of Dynamic Psychotherapy: Free Association

"Say whatever comes to mind." It may seem like a simple request, but once we begin, we find that our mind is not so easily or freely expressed! The *method* of psychodynamic therapy is called free association. It involves allowing the flow of thoughts to be expressed verbally, without editing or omitting those that may seem unacceptable. Allowing thoughts to flow freely into words without restricting or judging these thoughts is a unique skill. When the client says whatever comes to mind, any and all thoughts can become grist for the therapeutic mill. The risk of free associating is that something shameful will rise to the surface. The client risks revealing all aspects—positive and negative—of herself to another. The client risks being who she truly is and facing that honestly, without the protection of denial or family-of-origin rules. What comes to mind can be studied for themes, symbolism, and unconscious conflicts. As the client talks, both she and the therapist observe the string of thoughts. They are looking for places where the client may be tempted to edit or criticize. They are looking for evidence of the unconscious.

How it Works: Working Through

Working through is a bit like wrestling with demons. The working-through process involves revisiting important psychic events. In revisiting, the therapist can accompany the client in forming new perspectives and identifying feelings that happened at the time. A deeper understanding of the event, its consequences and lingering effects, may free the client from repeating old patterns of coping. This process takes time, as the ego releases memories for work at its own self-protective pace. Places in development that were traumatic can be revisited, feelings validated, and perspectives clarified. Through a reexamination of the traumatic periods or events, the client is able to free psychic energy that is tied up in containing anxieties associated with the conflicts.

The process of working through involves identifying conflicting feelings about an issue or event. Unconscious wishes or fantasies are observed to understand better the mental forces at play. Consequences of these mental forces are observed. The act of verbally expressing elements of the conflict may provide relief through the process of emotional catharsis. Catharsis is a relief of anxiety through expression of emotions and thoughts. Once these elements of the conflict are illuminated, the client can operate with a fuller awareness of his motives. Choices about new behaviors and reactions can be implemented. Old wishes can be released. Fears can be faced and reality embraced.

Resolving Conflicts

Increased awareness and understanding the conscious and unconscious elements of conflict can allow for a resolution of them. Through the method of free association, you can investigate the unconscious forces that maintain certain conflicts and anxieties. For example, if a client has experienced early loss and abandonment, present-day relationships might be affected by those atavistic fears and anxieties. There may be undue anxiety about time spent together in relationships, or resentment at not being included in relationships with peers. As early conflicts are better understood, it is possible to see how they might be reenacted or repeated in currrent situations. The forces that keep these patterns in place might include unfulfilled wished for gratification, such as a longing for love. Or anger that was unable to be expressed at the time may need to be recognized before it can be relinquished.

Insight

When you begin to develop an understanding of your true inner self, it is called insight. Insight is really just awareness. It comes about through the process of observation and understanding. The therapist uses his understanding of the mind and pays careful attention to your words and behaviors in order to offer suggestions that might produce insight into your feelings or behaviors. With insight comes choice, and therefore change. As I understand why I feel and act as I do, I can make changes in my situation or in myself. Insight produces freedom from the prison of repeating old patterns.

Making the Unconscious Conscious

One purpose of psychodynamic psychotherapy is to increase awareness of unconscious functioning. Freud suggested that only a small part of mental life is accessible through normal conscious awareness. Dreams have been called the "royal road to the unconscious." Dynamic therapy might include the analysis of dreams, as the client explores his unconscious activity by discussing, observing, and understanding dreams with the therapist.

Understanding the meaning of dreams must be individualized. There are no useful dream symbols cookbooks that can be used to interpret your dreams. The meanings of dream events and symbols must be interpreted in light of individual personality and life experience. Dreams must be understood within the continuity of your mind and experience. Certain censors that influence waking consciousness are removed during dream activity. Opposites may have the same meaning; for example, no may mean yes, and yes may mean no. Fears are also wishes. Something dreamed in the negative may be a disowned part of the self but a part of the self nonetheless.

Remembering dreams can be enhanced by dream work. Some clinicians recommend keeping a notebook by the bedside, and writing a stream-of-consciousness paragraph immediately upon awakening. Simply telling yourself you want to remember dreams upon awakening may bring increased awareness. Remembering dreams may be influenced by foods, drugs, and alcohol.

Interpreting the meaning of dreams is a highly personalized process. Symbols in dreams can arise from multiple sources. One source is bodily sensations. For example, if someone experiences the urge to urinate at night, dreams may contain an image of running water. Or, if someone is hungry, a dream may contain a hollow tunnel.

Dreams must be placed in the continuity of mental life. It seems as if dreams are alien to ourselves, disowned or cut off. Dreams may contain impulses that are warded off during conscious awareness. However, as much as a dream may seem uncharacteristic of the dreamer, it is a product of the dreamer's mind. Understanding the continuity of mental life provides a context for dream symbols. For example, if a person dreams of a desk, it may be because she sits at a desk all day at work. Recent conscious mind activity is available to the mind as it dreams. Events and interactions with people may be incorporated into dream symbols.

Transference and Countertransference

Some symptoms arise because of a fundamental unconscious repetition of early relationships. Our earliest relationships form the basis for our social approach to the world. As adults, we may often unconsciously repeat these relationships either because they were satisfying originally or because we wish to correct some disappointment. This has been called the transference of everyday life. We have a tendency to see others as they fit into our early dramas. When we look for certain characteristics, we find them. For example, if our early care givers were authoritarian, we may have a tendency to view relationships with teachers as based on authority, even though the teacher may be quite egalitarian. When the teacher offers a suggestion, we see it as evidence of being authoritarian. There is a distortion in the relationship, which does not allow for the full experience of present-day reality.

Most people who participate in therapy develop strong feelings about their therapist, although, as with any relationship, the longer the duration, the most intense and complex feelings become. Clients are often surprised and embarrassed about the intensity of feelings that develop and may be reluctant to discuss them openly. For example, a client may notice increasing feelings of dependency and look forward with anticipation and excitement to meetings. Do not be afraid to discuss feelings such as these with your therapist. It is important to understand these feelings in context. They are valuable to the therapy process and will help you better understand important aspects of psychological functioning.

As in everyday life, elements of early relationships are played out in the relationship between client and therapist. The client gives meaning to the therapist's verbalizations and behaviors. How a client interprets their therapist's responses involves the mechanism of projection. It is as if the therapist's neutral presentation becomes a blank screen, ready to receive direction and form from the client's expectations. For example, if the therapist is slow to sit down at the beginning of each session, the client may interpret this as lack of interest. The therapist may in actuality have a bad back and deliberately uses slow movements to minimize discomfort when sitting.

The projections of these expectations onto the therapist are extremely valuable. Because the therapist has good self-awareness, she can tell when the client is reacting to a characteristic that is not hers. The therapist can question the client about the distortions in the relationship, and together they can study the projections. This allows the client to view clearly how relationships are distorted, and can free contemporary relationships from these early constrictions. For example, if a client experienced early family life that involved frequent arguments, as an adult, he may argue frequently with significant others. A belief that couples argue is unconsciously reenacted. If the client attempts to reenact this pattern with a therapist, the therapist may be aware of frequent loss of his neutral stance. The pattern of arguing can be understood as belonging to an earlier time, and release of the belief that couples argue may free the client to relate in a more cooperative way with significant others.

Countertransference

Countertransference involves the biases and projections that the therapist brings to the therapy independent of the client. For example, if a therapist has had negative experiences with early care givers who had excessive dependency needs, the therapist may have difficulty tolerating the needs of the client. This has nothing to do with the client and is not a reflection of anything excessive on the client's part. It is a limitation in the therapist as a result of his personal history. Countertransference feelings may develop as a result of interactions in the psychotherapy process. For example, if a client has transference feelings that project the therapist as critical and harshly judgmental, the therapist may unconsciously identify with these expectations and find himself being unusually harsh and critical.

The key to coping with transference and countertransference is self-awareness. Ideally, the therapist has been analyzed, so that the effect of his personality on the therapy process can be minimized. If the therapist is aware of unconscious tendencies, he is less likely to interfere with the natural development of projection. Through the process of psychotherapy, the client develops the powers of self-observation. The client can begin to identify inappropriate remnants from earlier experiences. As the therapist and client together look for distortions in the relationship, a clearer understanding of motivations in the relationship is achieved. Naturally, the ultimate goal is to be able to relate to individuals as they are in reality, without distortions that interfere with their genuine self-expression. For example, a client may have a historical tendency to deny feelings of anger in self and others. When this tendency is brought into awareness, significant others will be freer to express feelings of anger without being minimized by the client.

Resistance

Resistance is inevitable in dynamic psychotherapy. Resistance involves the mind's forces that resist change and growth. These forces may manifest in behaviors such as missed payments, missed appointments, or even forgetting to bring important events into the therapy. Although the client may consciously desire insight and change, as therapy progresses, anxiety about change can be aroused. This anxiety is a warning that elements formerly banished to the unconscious may be threatening to emerge into consciousness. When these distressing awarenesses begin to become conscious, anxiety threatens to disrupt your work of psychotherapy.

It is also natural to have something therapists call resistance or feelings of not wanting to participate in therapy. Resistance is not necessarily a reason to stop treatment. Resistance is an illusion created by the mind to protect the status quo and frustrate change. It is important to acknowledge feelings of resistance but not necessarily to respond by changing decisions or behaviors. It's a bit like not wanting to go to school in the morning as a child. Of course we need to go because we have things to learn.

Termination

Eventually, the time will come when the process of therapy will end. Under ideal circumstances, therapy has gone on long enough for you to reach your goals. The decision to end formal sessions is ideally mutual, coming initially from the client but supported by the therapist. The client may feel satisfied that there is a congruence between the private and public self. The client may have developed an increased self-awareness and is now able to identify the impact of unconscious forces, as well as minimize their effects. The client may have developed an appreciation for the varied aspects of mental functioning and has a sense of self-acceptance.

It has been said that the goal of psychotherapy is to turn misery into common ordinary unhappiness. This is a significant accomplishment for the client who no longer experiences misery. It would be unreasonable to expect psychotherapy to be able to eradicate all feelings of unhappiness. Ordinary life involves ups and downs. Unhappy moments are bound to occur. These unhappy feelings serve to make feelings of happiness all the more precious and valuable.

So when the client and therapist agree, a final meeting date will be set. It is not unusual to experience an increase in anxiety as the date for termination approaches. Often, the symptoms that caused the initiation of treatment may recur temporarily. It is as if the client is saying to the therapist, "See, I still need you!" The termination should not necessarily be postponed because of this distress. Rather, a period of evaluation should be attempted to see if the client is indeed able to suspend treatment. The right to return to treatment if needed should be reserved.

The therapist also experiences a loss at the termination of therapy. If the relationship has lasted for a significant time, the importance of the relationship may be illustrated by feelings of loss. The therapist's goal is to become obsolete. Like a good-enough parent, the therapist should expect the client to develop coping skills that facilitate autonomy. Launching a client from a successful psychotherapy is a metaphorical birth, and the therapist plays the role of midwife. The goal is a healthy separation that produces an autonomous individual capable of interdependence and emotional well-being.

The client will undoubtedly carry in his mind a mental representation of the therapist. The client may have become used to consulting with this mental image between sessions. Clients frequently say, "I thought of what you would say," referring to the therapist's characteristic style of responding. This introject may be a permanent resource for some clients, adding to the history of personal relationships that contributes to blueprints and patterns of relating.

CHAPTER 7

Behavioral and Cognitive Therapy

Behavioral Therapy

Behavioral therapy, which evolved out of a traditionally American approach to psychology, involves action. Whereas European psychoanalysts focused on unconscious mental forces, American psychologists originally concentrated on observable and measurable behaviors. Through observation and measurement of behaviors in animals and humans, and laboratory experiments, behaviorists developed the theory that personality is acquired primarily through learned experiences. Behaviorists believe that we come into the world as blank slates, equal to one another. They believe that as we encounter experiences, we learn ways to respond to the challenges by trial and error, and by experiencing consequences. Behavioral theory, also called learning theory, suggests that through rewards and punishments, learning takes place, and human personality is shaped. This view of psychology was readily accepted in American culture because of our fondness for the belief that all people are created equal and that life is what you make of it. Behaviorists and Americans like to believe that given the right circumstances, anyone can become a success.

Behaviorists first concentrated on understanding the relationship between stimulus and response. They observed that stimuli become associated with certain types of responses or behaviors. Pairing is the process that occurs when events happen together in time. If a shock is delivered when a white light is turned on, the white light will become associated with pain. This is also called classical conditioning. In a more complex example, if a high school student is ridiculed (or given negative feedback) by the teacher every time she comes to class, the student will feel badly about herself each time she goes to school. Feeling badly about oneself might become associated with being in school. The behaviorist believes this is because of actual rewards or punishments in the environment, not because of unconscious mental forces.

Skinner, a well known behavioral psychologist, demonstrated the principles of conditioning in a well-known experiment that involved a toddler named Albert and a white rabbit. Dr. Skinner presented Albert with a harmless white rabbit, and at the same time, introduced a loud noise that startled and frightened the child. Soon, Albert became frightened just at the sight of the white rabbit, demonstrating learning, or a change in behavior, through association and pairing. Interestingly, this response was found to generalize to other stimuli. Albert became frightened of any furry white animal, such as a rat or a white kitten.

Early behaviorists focused only on stimulus and response, and failed to take into account individual differences in the human organism, which modifies how we respond to various situations. For example, not all of us respond the same way to a given stimulus. Behaviorists began to take into account the processing that goes on inside an individual, and started to study the stimulus-organism-response equation.

This type of learning is known as operant conditioning. In these situations, more than a simple pairing of stimulus and response is required. Some behavior, or individual processing, on the part of the subject is necessary to elicit a desired consequence or response. For example, pigeons can be taught to press levers (a behavior on the environment) or select colored lights when food is presented as a reward. Both humans and animals will naturally work to perform behaviors that result in positive rewards or avoid painful consequences.

Behaviorists have studied patterns and schedules of reinforcements to see how learning can be most effective. They have found that the strongest reinforcement for repeated behavior is when rewards come on a random schedule. We tend to work harder for a consequence when we know that eventually our desired response will occur. For example, if a slot machine pays out randomly rather than on a time schedule or based on the number of times the lever is pulled, we tend to stay with the activity.

Changes involve acquiring new behaviors or extinguishing old habits. The process of shaping involves providing rewards as a client gradually acquires a desired behavior. For example, if the goal is to walk across the floor, each step is rewarded, and the desired behavior is reinforced.

Punishments don't alter behaviors as much as we would think. Decreasing a habit can better be accomplished by withholding rewards rather than by inflicting painful punishments. Punishments can have unintended consequences. We have all heard about a child who repeats an undesirable behavior because "negative attention is better than no attention at all."

Noted psychologist Albert Bandura contributed a useful concept to learning theory when he discovered that we do not necessarily need to experience all situations ourselves in order to learn. He noted that even animals can learn by watching the behavior of others. He called this phenomenon observational learning. We can watch other people's behaviors, and the consequences, and learn from their experiences rather than needing to experience everything ourselves. Because of this, modeling can be an effective method of altering behavior. Modeling literally means showing by example. For example, a therapist might model effective problem solving for the client by actually solving a problem in the session.

Behavioral approaches to therapy involve activities and actual real-life experiences. These therapies differ from purely talking forms of treatment and incorporate learning through doing. Sometimes just talking about problems is not enough. Insight does not necessarily produce changes in behavior. For example, one client was addicted to cigarettes for many years. She could discuss in great detail that this habit represented unconscious self-destructive tendencies, a fixation on oral gratification, and a defense against anxiety. Talking about wanting to quit did not stop her from smoking. In the end, she needed to take action and change actual behaviors in order to resolve this addiction. She needed to actually alter habits and experience being a nonsmoker; not just talk about or under-stand the symptom. Sometimes, we need to feel and live a change in real life.

Behavioral therapies are most useful for clients who enjoy active collaboration. If a person's natural style is to act on be-haviors, an active, behavioral form of working through may be most appropriate. People who are action-oriented may find be-havior therapy more in concert with their personal style. Peo-ple who express emotions through actions rather than words may find the introspection of psychodynamic therapy tedious and unproductive. People with anxiety disorders have good re-sults with relaxation training and response prevention. Re-ward economies and social-skills training have been shown to be effective for clients with schizophrenia. Behavioral thera-pies are designed to help clients learn new responses that are more adaptive.

Now let me present several techniques used in behavioral therapies.

Relaxation Training

Stress is everywhere. We have recently realized that many of life's physical and emotional problems are stress related. Stress plays an enormous role in psychological and physiological well-being, and reducing it is a skill we can learn and practice. Anxiety can be managed through practicing specific techniques learned in a behavioral therapy. Learning how to relax can be an enjoyable and rewarding practice. By learning to minimize experiences of stress and controlling occurrences of stress, we can significantly improve our lives.

Our human nervous system is set up to help us cope with danger by using fight or flight responses. One part of the nervous system, the sympathetic branch, helps us gear up and get ready to run or fight. It releases adrenaline and promotes blood flow to areas of the body needed when an active response is required. Another part of the nervous system, the parasympathetic branch, helps us calm down after encountering danger. The parasympathetic system helps us slow down, releases relaxing hormones, and reroutes blood flow to internal vital organs. The parasympathetic and sympathetic nervous systems cannot operate simultaneously. When we activate the parasympathetic system, we calm down.

Breathing is the key to the parasympathetic nervous system. Eastern health systems, such as Ayurveda and traditional Chinese medicine, have long recognized the importance of breathing. In Ayurveda, the practice of yoga involves breathing techniques to promote health and relaxation. In China, the practice of t'ai chi and *chi quong* use breath work. Recently, Western medicine has recognized the benefits of working with the breath to induce relaxation. Dr. Andrew Weil at the University of Arizona says, "If you think you're breathing deeply enough, you're not."

Promoting relaxation through deep breathing is easy and can be practiced anywhere, anytime. Whenever you feel over-stressed, take three deep breaths, fully expanding your diaphragm. When you are breathing deeply, you should feel your abdomen expand, your ribs expand to the side, and your chest rise. Breathe in for a count of seven, hold for a count of three, and then fully release all your breath to a count of eight. You may wish to breathe in through your nose and breathe out making a soft *ch* sound in the back of your throat.

Working with your breathing is the simplest form of relaxation training. Other techniques for relaxation include visualization, guided imagery, and self-hypnosis. These techniques involve quieting the mind, achieving a relaxed state, and focusing on images that promote positive feelings. Some people are wary of entering a state of hypnosis because of the types of theatrical performances associated with this term. Hypnosis is, in essence, simply a profoundly relaxed state. While under, you are aware of your surroundings, can easily awaken, and cannot be made to behave in ways that you would not ordinarily do. If you are working with a therapist who is trained in hypnosis, he can guide you into a relaxed state by helping you focus your awareness. There are also many high-quality commercially available audiotapes that can be used to practice relaxation through imagery and self-hypnosis.

If you want to try this experience, begin by sitting quietly and focusing on your breath. Just observe your breathing and begin to relax into a comfortable position. Think about relaxing every muscle, from the top of your head to the tips of your toes. With each breath, you take in calm, with each breath out, you release tension. Focus on relaxing the muscles in your face, neck, back, and arms. Relax your abdomen and legs with each breath. Once you feel comfortable and relaxed, think of a place where you have felt a profound sense of well-being. It may be a beach by the ocean, or a forest with a running stream. Imagine the details of your special place. Notice how comfortable you feel. Stay in your relaxed place, noticing the details and the positive feelings. When you are ready, you can return from your place with several deep breaths, feeling refreshed and as if you have had a long nap.

This is a simplified version of self-hypnosis or visualization. You can work on a personalized exercise with your therapist. Ask her to make an audiotape of the session for you to use at home. Although relaxation through imagery is helpful for most people, some who are highly anxious cannot use this particular technique successfully. If this type of exercise makes you feel nervous about letting your guard down, a progressive muscle-relaxation technique might be more helpful.

Progressive muscle relaxation involves tensing and releasing all the muscle groups in your body. For example, begin by tensing the muscles in your forehead, holding them for a count of five, then releasing and smoothing the muscles. Then tense and release your neck muscles. Move on to your shoulders, then your arms, hands, and so on. Tense and hold each group of muscles, then release and smooth as you breathe out and relax. Progressive muscle relaxation is different from guided imagery and hypnosis in that it does not require you to wander around in your imagination. It works with the physical sensations of tensing and releasing muscles.

Autogenic Training

Autogenic means self-regulation. Autogenic training is related to yoga and hypnosis. This technique involves learning skills that are designed to counteract the natural fight or flight response of the nervous system. The therapist will help you develop an inner dialogue that concentrates on feeling heaviness in the extremities; warmth; slower breathing and heart rate;

and a cooling in the forehead. For example, get comfortable, then begin concentrating feeling your limbs growing heavy. Say to yourself, "My right arm is heavy," "My abdomen is warm," "My heart rate is slowing." Practice this two to three times a day, as self-regulation is achieved through regular practice of these exercises.

Biofeedback

Biofeedback is a specialized form of relaxation training that involves monitoring several physical parameters, including heart rate and blood pressure, while learning to attain a relaxed state through hypnosis or visualization. As the client masters relaxation techniques, he can begin to develop conscious control of these physical parameters. Through biofeedback, he learns to reduce blood pressure and heart rate as a part of anxiety and stress management.

Biofeedback is widely used, and treatments are frequently reimbursed by third-party payers. However, studies suggest that the effectiveness of biofeedback training has no additional benefit over simple relaxation training alone. Using machinery to demonstrate physical changes is unnecessary, and mastery over physical manifestations of stress can be achieved through relaxation training alone. Fees for biofeedback may be higher than for relaxation training because of the high-tech appearance of the machinery used to monitor physical parameters.

Systematic Desensitization

Systematic desensitization involves learning the relaxation response or relaxation techniques, then using these techniques while gradually exposing the client to the feared stimulus.

Exposure can be either through the imagination, in vivo, or real life. The rationale for this type of therapy is that the central nervous system simply cannot be relaxed and anxious at the same time. The client achieves a relaxed state, then imagines or actually exposes herself to the feared object or situation. If she notices any anxiety symptoms, she returns to the relaxation process, decreasing attention to the object of fear. Gradually, the client experiences mastery over a feared situation or object.

Symptoms-Based Exercises

Exercises designed to address specific symptoms may be used as an intervention in behavioral therapy. The therapist and client actively collaborate to design exercises individually tailored to address specific symptoms constellations. Exercises may involve practicing new behaviors to allow the client to have a more adaptive response to anxiety.

Response prevention is a technique that involves deliberately inhibiting a maladaptive response. For example, if a client with germ phobias and a compulsion to wash her hands frequently comes for behavioral treatment, a response-prevention exercise may be practiced. When the client comes into contact with the germ stimulus, she is prevented from washing by being placed in an environment where no washing is possible.

Symptoms substitution is another behavioral technique designed to extinguish maladaptive symptoms. For example, if a client has a tendency to act out anger by breaking objects, he might, with the assistance of a therapist, instead walk or run to dissipate the feelings of anger.

In its earlier forms, specific behavioral techniques were applied to selected symptoms regardless of the function of that symptom in personality. More recent applications of behavioral therapy involve application of techniques in a way that is consistent with dynamic psychological functions. The meaning of the symptom is understood from a dynamic perspective. Then a more adaptive behavior that can perform the same function as the original symptomatic behavior is substituted. Therapy is more likely to be effective because the dynamic forces of the mind have been considered.

Reward Economics

A reward economy involves setting up an environment that rewards desired behaviors, and at times punishes undesirable behavioral responses. This therapy is based on principles of operant conditioning and attempts to reinforce specific stimulus and responses. The idea behind reward economies is that behaviors that elicit rewards are likely to be repeated, and behaviors that are not rewarded or are punished won't be.

Schedules of rewards have been studied in great detail. Understanding the influence of rewards and punishments on behaviors calls for us to look at the person. Interestingly, human beings tend to work harder to receive a reward that is given on an inconsistent schedule, such as with a slot machine.

For a token economy to be effective, the environment must offer consistent reinforcement. If a token economy is used in a school, all the teachers must implement the program. This type of intervention is useful for clients who need external structure and support. A written agreement of expected behaviors and rewards or consequences is often developed in order to make expectations clear. Token economies have been used with clients who have mental retardation and autism, and has even had some success with schizophrenia. The key for success is to personalize behaviors and rewards to the individual client. The therapist must design rewards that are specifically gratifying for the individual client.

Behavioral Contracting

At times, the client and therapist may find it helpful to enter into a written agreement about what will happen in therapy. Drafting such an agreement provides an opportunity to clarify expectations and consequences. For example, if a therapist is working with someone who is thinking about suicide, they might write down a plan of action to be followed in case these thoughts occur. The client might agree to call the therapist before acting on these impulses. In exchange, the therapist might agree to be available to the client on an emergency basis, by long-range paging. Consequences of acting on these impulses rather than calling for help can be identified in advance so that the client understands what will happen. For example, the client understands that the therapist will suspend outpatient sessions until the behavior is under control.

Contracts might also involve agreements about what will happen in therapy. For example, if a client is attempting to reach a specific goal, such as decreasing aggressive behavior, an agreement about rewards for achieving this goal might be identified. The client might be able to choose some specific reward for refraining from acting on these impulses.

Cognitive Therapy

There has been a long-standing argument in the field of psychology about what comes first: the thought or the feeling. Do thoughts determine feelings or do feelings determine thoughts? Do we feel an emotion, then label it with a thought, or do our thoughts give rise to patterns or memories of emotions? For example, do we see a gray sky, think gray sky, think/remember depressed feelings associated with rain, then feel depressed because we see a gray sky? Or do we notice a disinterest or heaviness, feeling blue or hopeless, remember these emotional experiences, and call it depression? The answer is probably both. Thoughts can trigger feelings, and feelings can trigger thoughts. In any event, it is clear that thoughts and feelings are inextricably intertwined.

Cognitive therapy has its conceptual roots in the computer age. Our models of the mind tend to be constructed according to the popular models of the time. In Freud's era, the engineering models of the time were hydraulic, as steam and combustion engines became widely used. His early models of the mind look at mental processing in terms of pressures and releases. Cognitive therapy follows our cultural development into the information-processing age. As we learn about bytes of data and memory-storage units in the computer and study models of artificial intelligence, theories of the mind evolve along similar lines. We began to view mental activity in terms of input, storage, retrieval, and output. Cognitive therapy looks at how we think and styles of information-processing, such as scanning and screening. These theories suggest that symptoms arise for maladaptive thought patterns.

Cognitive therapy involves working with thoughts. We are always thinking, planning, daydreaming, and worrying. The focus of cognitive therapy is on how we think, what patterns and situations produce our thoughts, and understanding the impact of these thoughts on emotions, coping, and personality. The process of cognitive therapy can increase your awareness of thought distortions and help you implement changes in thinking. Exercises that may involve observing and altering your behaviors may be prescribed.

You can easily see the impact of thoughts on feelings by trying a small experiment. Try thinking repeatedly, "I am a capable, well-liked person," or some other positive affirmation. See how you feel in a half hour. Now think about all those times you said to yourself, "That was stupid," or "I can't do that," or "I look fat," and begin to develop an awareness of how this critical diatribe makes you feel. Unfortunately, we internalize our critics who taught us all that socialized behavior, like using a toilet and getting good grades. If critics have been harsh, we will be harsh with ourselves. Cognitive therapy involves monitoring for distortions in thinking, then correcting any dysfunctional thoughts. Working with thoughts can clearly have emotional benefits.

Cognitive therapy has been found to be particularly successful in treating depression and anxiety. In his book *Feeling Good,* David Burns, M.D., a psychiatrist at the University of Pennsylvania, guides the reader through the cognitive-analysis process and identifies methods for combating depression. Typically, when a client is depressed, an internal dialogue develops, which disparages the client, the world, and the future. By observing and altering this dialogue, the client can achieve significant emotional relief. For example, if a client is repeatedly saying to herself, "Nothing good ever happens to me," she is unlikely to identify experiences that do have benefit. If she actively changes her mantra to something like, "Good things can happen for me," the likelihood of drawing positive experiences increases.

Beck's Cognitive Triad

Nationally known cognitive psychiatrist Aaron Beck, M.D., suggests three cognitive factors that form the foundation of our well-being: Our view of our *self,* the *world,* and the *future* has a profound impact on our adaptation, thinking, and feeling. For example, if we view ourselves as capable of solving most of life's problems, we will more likely attempt to resolve challenges that confront us. If we believe that we can influence the outcome of events in our lives through our actions, we will feel empowered to take corrective actions. If we view the world as a just and fair place, we are more likely to have a basic sense of trust about life events. If we are hopeful about the future, we will be better able to endure different circumstances. On the other hand, if we believe ourselves to be helpless victims and that the world is basically unfair and always presenting insurmountable obstacles, we are likely to feel depressed. If we feel incapable of influencing the outcome through our own actions, the future is likely to seem hopeless.

Common Distortions

Several common thought-pattern distortions have been identified. These include catastrophizing, personalizing, and all-or-none thinking. Catastrophizing involves a perspective of the worst-possible scenario in everyday life. Have you ever heard someone say, "This is the worst day of my life!" or "I'll just die if he doesn't call," or "I'm finished if I fail this test!"? This is catastrophizing. It involves blowing up consequences of ordinary events into catastrophic proportions. It is not the end of the world if you get a traffic ticket, bounce a check, or these days, are arrested! We love people who recover. In life, there are few true catastrophes.

Personalizing is a common distortion, which involves relating everything that happens to yourself. For example, if your boss doesn't say "good morning" you may begin thinking, "He doesn't like me" or "I've done something wrong," when the truth is that the boss didn't have time for breakfast and is thinking of hunger pangs, not morning greetings.

All-or-none thinking happens when you have a tendency to see things in black or white terms. Life would be simpler if events and people fit neatly into simple categories: all good or all bad. For example, "I didn't get the promotion, I am a bad employee," or "I have to buy that house or I will be a failure." Dogmatic thinking that does not allow for specific alterations may be the all or none, "All teachers are good," "All dogs are bad," etc. Reality is much more complex, and every situation has many shades of gray.

Rational Emotive Therapy

Nationally known cognitive psychologist Albert Ellis suggests that irrational beliefs are at the heart of psychological symptoms. He developed a method of influencing these faulty perceptions, called Rational Emotive Therapy. This theory suggests that a person's value system and beliefs interpret certain experiences negatively and therefore produce emotional distress. The symptoms are caused by the beliefs about an event rather than the event itself. If we can identify the underlying irrational beliefs that are causing us to negatively interpret an event, we can correct the misinterpretation and feel better. Ellis finds evidence for these beliefs by studying the *self-talk* that goes on in a person's thinking.

Some of the irrational beliefs he identified include:

_____ It is absolutely necessary for me to be loved and approved of by nearly every person with whom I have close contact.

_____ I must be thoroughly competent and adequate in all respects, or I am worthless.

_____ If things are not the way I like them to be, it is a terrible catastrophe.

_____ Unhappiness is caused by external events over which I have almost no control.

_____ Some things are terribly dangerous and life-threatening, so I must keep thinking about them most of the time. I should be very upset over other people's problems and disturbances.

—— There is always a right and precise solution to human problems, and if that is not found, I must be very upset. (See Sundberg, Taplin, and Tyler, 1983.)

In addition to techniques for working with general psychological difficulties, Ellis offered a rational approach to recovery from addictions. In his work, *Rational Recovery,* Ellis removes the aspect of a higher power from the twelve steps and creates rational steps toward recovery. Using this approach, addiction behavior is seen as based on irrational thinking. Irrational thoughts keep the alcoholic drinking. Rational thoughts can get and keep the alcoholic sober. Members embrace rationality rather than using references to a higher power.

Thought Stopping

Thought stopping has been found to be useful for people who tend to ruminate or obsess about certain thoughts. It is a simple but effective technique for altering unwanted, recurrent cognitions. This technique involves concentrating on the unwanted thoughts, then, suddenly, you stop thinking these thoughts and empty your mind. The sudden stop can be accompanied by saying or thinking, "Stop!" Stopping can be reinforced with either a loud noise or snapping a rubber band that is kept around the wrist. The rationale for thought stopping is that the unpleasant or sudden stimulus will interrupt unpleasant, unwanted thoughts and be replaced by a more positive quiet or emptiness.

Assertiveness Training

All of us are able to be assertive in some situations. In other situations, we may become passive or aggressive. Assertiveness training teaches people to express themselves more effectively in a variety of situations. These methods assume that non-assertive behaviors come from mistaken assumptions. Mistaken assumptions can be refuted with a cognitive reminder about your rights in any situation. For example, many people are taught growing up that it is selfish to put your own needs first. This can be corrected by remembering that in some situations you have a legitimate right to put your needs first.

The process of assertiveness training involves practice in identifying the three types of behaviors: aggressive, assertive, and passive. Then you select a situation in which you wish to be more assertive. You describe problem responses and identify how you would like to change. You can write a script for the situation, which includes a reminder of your legitimate rights and I messages. You can plan your body language and practice it with the therapist. You can practice eye contact, posture, speech, and gestures. Assertiveness training helps you look for win-win situations and avoid being manipulated.

Cognitive Behaviorist Approaches

During the 1970s a synthesis of behavioral and cognitive approaches began to occur. Behaviorists began to embrace ideas about the impact of information processing on outward actions. Albert Bandura advanced the theory by discovering that we can learn through observation and modeling.

One well-known cognitive behaviorist Donald Meichenbaum has focused treatment on acquisition of cognitive, social, and behavioral skills. These methods involve developing specific thoughts that can guide an individual through a desired behavior. It is a way to develop self-talk that supports the desired outcome. Meichenbaum first developed techniques for self-instruction to assist hyperactive children in controlling their behaviors. By giving yourself specific cognitive suggestions and instructions, your coping abilities will improve. It is a way to talk yourself through a problem. For example, when working on a difficult math problem, you might say to yourself, "Relax, you are developing improved math skills; this is a learning process. Take your time, figure out which elements of the problem are to be worked with first. Which elements of the problem are irrelevant distractors? Break down the problem. You are a good student."

Another cognitive behavioral application was developed by George Spivak and Myrna Shurt at Hahnemann University in Philadelphia. Called interpersonal cognitive problem solving, the technique involves teaching types of thinking to facilitate successful problem solving. For example, the client might be taught how to think through consequences of behavioral choices before actually making the choice. These methods have recently been implemented with children in a wide range of prevention programs. If we can teach our children how to problem solve in a number of different ways, they are more likely to grow to become effectively coping adults and feel a sense of mastery. Spivak and Shure suggest that in order to help a child develop effective thinking, parents and teachers can dialogue with children about the following issues: See how the child views the problem in a way that is nonjudgmental. Be matter-of-fact and ask the child why he acted as he did. Talk to the child about how he feels and how others might have felt. Encourage him to suggest ways of dealing with the problem. Ask him to think about what might happen next. Generate and evaluate more than one solution.

Cognitive and behavioral therapies offer an important path toward the resolution of a variety of difficulties. For some people, it may be helpful to use these approaches either alternately or in conjunction with psychodynamic techniques. The lines that separate these therapies in theory are much less clear when working in a real-life clinical situation. For example, one client might use behavioral techniques, including relaxation, to stop self-destructive behaviors such as smoking, and then use a dynamic process to resolve underlying conflicts. A client in a psychodynamic therapy might spent time looking at irrational thoughts in order to correct distortions and use free association to uncover the importance of early life experiences.

Although blending different techniques may be helpful for the client, studies suggest that therapists who embrace one form of therapy wholeheartedly tend to have better outcomes than therapists who attempt to practice from an eclectic approach.

CHAPTER 8

Biological Therapies

Pharmacotherapy

Since ancient times, the treatment of health problems has involved the use of medicinal preparations. Traditional healers recommended combinations of herbs. Chinese and Indian systems of healing have employed the use of herbs for thousands of years. Contemporary physicians, trained with an emphasis on prescribing, combine the use of naturally occurring and synthetic medications. As consumers, we have available to us a vast array of medication choices.

Medications should never be taken lightly. They have a profound impact on the human system. It is important for anyone who uses medication to obtain as much information as needed to make fully informed choices, as well as to fully understand the effects of any medication choices. This involves developing a basic understanding of physical functioning and clinical problems, as well as the impact of therapeutic agents. Information about these topics is easily obtained by asking your professional care providers. They expect to teach as a part of the services they provide.

As a rule, it is best to take any medication only when necessary. Nature has constructed an amazing self-restoring, adaptive, developing organism in the human body. We are capable of regenerating and restoring homeostasis. As the tradition of nursing suggests, healing takes place best when the environment optimally supports these natural processes. This means allowing for rest, clean air, sunlight, therapeutic nutrition, effective drainage, balanced activities, and peace of mind. When the environment allows for therapeutic conditions, the human organism is often capable of restoring its own optimal functioning.

In addition to using these general techniques, we have a huge selection of pharmaceutical agents available to alleviate both symptoms and diseases. As a society we are captivated with the idea of the magic bullet. We share a delusion that we will ultimately stumble on that single substance that will correct all ills. We target specific aspects of a disease process, whether genetic or chemical. Other systems of healing tended to take the whole human organism into account, working to understand how parts of the system function together. As consumers, advertisements regularly remind us of the benefits of over-the-counter products. We are encouraged to take compounds to relieve pain, promote sleep, decrease gastric upset, and suppress allergies. Before deciding to take one of these preparations, it may be helpful to view symptoms as information. Your body provides feedback about how things are going, either by functioning smoothly or by sending distress signals. Symptoms such as headache, insomnia, and indigestion may be alerting you to some necessary life-style change. This is so important it must be repeated: Symptoms are information that alerts you to the need for *life-style change*. Whenever possible, it is best to attend to these symptoms by making adjustments in self-care behaviors, such as increasing rest, exercise, or changing diet. Pharmacological interventions can be harsh and have a tendency to produce dramatic side effects. They should be used judiciously.

However, the realities of life in these pressured times often require that we continue to function despite the appearance of symptoms. Pharmacological interventions can produce quick, powerful results. Nonpharamcologic options for treating distress are not always readily available (such as a massage, or the ability to sleep). It is natural to want immediate relief from uncomfortable symptoms. When we want quick relief, we can and do choose to use medications.

It is important to weigh the potential benefits and risks of any medication. Let's look at the choices involved in headache remedies. Although acetaminophen promises to relieve most headaches in standard doses, it is metabolized by the liver and can stress that organ's functioning. Aspirin also relieves headaches, but it can cause a tendency to bleed. Nonsteroidal anti-inflammatory agents also relieve headaches, but they can cause gastric distress. If the potential benefit of taking a medication clearly outweighs the potential risk, we must choose between pharmaceutical options.

For all medications, and most herbs, every action has a reaction. All medicines have intended and *unintended* effects. Unwanted side effects must be recognized and considered in medication choices. For example, an antidepressant may decrease feelings of fatigue, but it may also suppress appetite. It may create dry mouth, constipation, or blurred vision.

Deciding which products are available without a prescription is a political/legal/economic process. Although the intent is to protect the well-being of the general public, it does not necessarily ensure that over-the-counter medications are "safe." Over-the-counter medications are powerful pharmacologic agents with potentially serious side effects. They should be taken in consultation with a health-care professional.

When you and your therapist find it appropriate, a prescription for medication may be considered. Prescription medications are designed to alleviate "target symptoms," and when used to treat specific conditions, can provide great relief. It is important to discuss fully any prescribed medication with the person issuing the prescription. Consumers should have a thorough understanding of the purpose of the medication, what effects and side effects can be expected, and how long the prescription is to be followed. Ask about restrictions of caffeine, alcohol, or food. Learn how and when to discontinue taking the prescription. Physicians, nurses, and pharmacists can provide detailed information, often in printed form. When more than one person is writing you prescriptions, it is essential that you tell them about all medications you're currently taking. Medications can interact with each other and have an antagonistic or potentiating effect. Pharmacologic substances are said to be *antagonistic* if they interfere with each other's intended effect. Medications that produce a stronger effect when taken in combination are said to *potentiate* each other.

Major Drug Classes

Psychoactive or psychotropic drugs are medications that have an impact on psychological functioning or mood. Many everyday substances have mood- and mind-altering properties. For example, coffee is a mood elevator and a mental stimulant. Alcohol is a sedative and slows mental processes. Since the mid 1950s, clinicians have been prescribing pharmacologic agents to alleviate emotional and cognitive symptoms. Several major drug classes will be discussed, including antidepressants, antianxiety agents, antipsychotics, and medications used to treat organic conditions.

Medications Used to Treat Mood Disorders

Three main types of drugs can be used to relieve symptoms of depression. These drugs alter blood levels of chemicals called neurotransmitters, which are thought to be involved in feelings of depression. The first antidepressant medications were tricyclic antidepressants, named after the structure of the chemical molecule. Tryclycic antidepressants include Amitriptyline (Elavil), Nortriptyline (Aventyl), Desipramine (Pamelor), Imipramine (Tofranil), and Protriptyline (Vicactil). These medications affect the neurotransmitter norepinephrine. These medications may be sedating and may help clients sleep better if taken before bed. The minor side effects of these drugs include constipation, dry mouth, and blurred vision. These medications may produce cardiac side effects and should not be used by clients with underlying heart disease or disorders.

A second type of antidepressants are the monoamine oxidase inhibitors. These include Marplan, Parnate, and Nardil. These drugs affect the amount of monoamines available at the neuronal synapses. These drugs are not particularly sedating, and may be most effective with depressions characterized by atypical symptoms. These medications will cause a serious, sudden rise in blood pressure if they mix with tyramine in the blood. Foods with large amounts of tyramines must be avoided by clients taking these medications. A strict diet that prohibits aged cheese, aged wine, bananas, chocolate, and alcohol must be followed. Research on an herbal monoamine oxidase inhibitor is beginning, as scientists study St. John's Wort.

A third group of antidepressants called selective serotonin re-uptake inhibitors has recently become popular. These medications made more serotonin available at the synapses in the brain. These medications may be activating and are best taken in the morning. They include Prozac, Zoloft, and Paxil. These antidepressants are popular because they have the least serious risk of side effects. They may create some nausea or restlessness. However, the risk of serious cardiac complications is reduced when compared with prior drug classes.

In addition to these major categories of antidepressants,

there are several atypical medications, including Desyrel and Doxepin. These drugs are also sedating and may improve sleep as well as mood.

The treatment of choice for bipolar or manic depression is lithium. Lithium has been shown to control episodes of mania and prevent the recurrence of manic and depressive episodes. Lithium has several side effects, including water retention and weight gain. Lithium levels must be monitored carefully in order to achieve a therapeutic dose. When lithium levels are too high, the client may experience nausea or vomiting, and may develop a fine tremor.

There are several medications in addition to lithium that can be used to help stabilize mood. Psychiatrists may prescribe Tegretol and Depakote to help someone with erratic mood swings.

Medications Used to Treat Anxiety

Antianxiety agents are sometimes called minor tranquilizers. Available since the early 1960s, benzodiazepines act directly on brain chemistry to alleviate feelings of anxiety. They also create feelings of well-being, and at higher doses may cause euphoria. Initially, these drugs were widely prescribed, but then it was discovered that they are highly addictive. They do have appropriate short-term use in certain groups of patients, such as someone with acute anxiety. Although there is some controversy about using these medications with the elderly, some clinicians find that if used cautiously, these medications can help the older adult with chronic anxiety. The first benzodiazepine was Valium. Additional drugs in this class include Ativan, Xanax, Serax, Tranxene, and Librium. Dalmane and Restoril are benzodiazepines used to treat insomnia. Each compound has a slightly different mix of sedation, euphoria, and antianxiety properties. The onset of effect, or how quickly each medication starts to work, is different. Recent trends favor the prescription of Klonopin (clonazepam), which is a longer-acting benzodiazepine that does not produce feelings of euphoria and holds less potential for abuse. Klonopin is often used in combination with other medications when there are more serious symptoms.

The long-term use of benzodiazepines is not generally recommended, as the central nervous system adjusts to the effects of these drugs, and sensations of anxiety may return. Or the client will require increasingly larger doses of the medication to achieve the desired effect. It is best to use these medications intermittently, giving the body a chance to recover between exposures to the drug.

Because these medications provide a sense of relaxation and occasionally, euphoria, clients who take them are at risk for developing a psychological dependency. When anxiety appears, it can become a coping mechanism to take a medication. Using this coping option can inhibit the development of more effective strategies that rely on strengthening intrapsychic mechanisms.

Buspar is a new antianxiety drug that has a gradual effect on anxiety symptoms. This medication may take several weeks to achieve the desired effect. It offers its most beneficial effects to clients who have not used benzodiazepines for anxiety management in the past. Clients who experience anxiety are uncomfortable. When a client with anxiety takes a benzodiazepine, relief is generally felt in a few minutes to an hour. For clients who have felt this relief, waiting the two to three weeks necessary for Buspar to take effect may be impossible. Buspar may be particularly useful for anxiety management in clients who have an addiction history and might become seriously dependent on benzodiazepines.

Beta-blockers such as Inderal inhibit physiological sensations that often accompany anxiety. The connection between physical signs of anxiety and an experience of psychological anxiety is interrupted. Beta-blockers are designed to lower blood pressure and slow the pulse. Increased pulse and blood pressure often accompany anxiety. The body begins to associate the feelings of increased pulse and blood pressure as evidence of anxiety, and thus may begin feeling anxious. When a client takes a beta-blocker, the physiological symptoms of anxiety are diminished, so the mind is less likely to interpret bodily sensations as the experience of anxiety.

Low-dose neuroleptics may also be used for clients with severe anxiety. Although these medications are traditionally used in higher doses in order to combat hallucinations, they may provide useful tranquilization in cases of anxiety. In low does, neuroleptics can slow thoughts to allow a client to organize and process information more effectively. They also have a sedative effect, which interferes with the perception of anxiety.

Medications Used to Treat Thought Disorders

The discovery of Thorazine in the mid 1950s was a significant breakthrough in the treatment of mental illness. When clients with severe mental illness took Thorazine, their behaviors improved. Hallucinations diminished in some clients, but significant improvement in activities of daily living were also noted. Significant numbers of clients who previously had to be institutionalized were able to leave the hospital and live in the community after taking this newly discovered medication. This drug class is sometimes called major tranquilizers. Later versions of neuroleptics include Navane, Prolixin, Stellazine, Trilafon, Mellaril, Haldol, Moban, and Loxitane. These medications all have serious side effects, including extrapyramidal symptoms, which involve sensations of restlessness, involuntary movements, or pacing. In addition, cholingeric effects of the medications include constipation, dry mouth, and blurred vision. In some clients, a permanent movement disorder that is essentially a Parkinson's syndrome can result from taking medications in this drug class. This side effect is called tardive dyskinesia, and may involve lip smacking, involuntary facial movements, pill rolling with the fingers, and a shuffling gait. Symptoms of movement disorders are now thought to be aggravated by changing the doses of these medications.

Recent developments in the pharmacological treatment of psychosis have given us several new agents to use. Clozaril was an exciting discovery because this new medication has a positive impact on the symptoms of schizophrenia without the risk of movement disorders. This drug was first marketed to treat clients who did not have a beneficial effect from traditional antipsychotics. It appears to have the most impact on the negative symptoms of schizophrenia and has engendered remarkable recovery in some. The negative symptoms include absence of ambition and drive, blunted emotional reactions, and decreased thoughts or feelings. However, Clozaril has a potentially life-threatening side effect: It may permanently eliminate the body's ability to produce white blood cells, which are responsible for immunity. This is called agranulocytosis. The number of clients who actually developed this side effect is small. However, the seriousness of this side effect requires that special precautions be taken for anyone on this medication. The drug cannot be prescribed unless clients have a weekly evaluation of white blood-cell counts. If a client develops any drop in white blood-cell production, the drug must be immediately discontinued. Again agranulocytosis is irreversible, so it must be monitored very closely. Another bothersome but not serious side effect of Clozaril is excessive saliva production. Clients may be bothered by nighttime drooling or the need for frequent swallowing.

New agents similar to Clozaril but without the serious adverse effects are being developed. For example, Resperidol reduces symptoms of psychosis but does not carry the risks to white blood-cell production. It has the benefits of limited side effects on the motor system.

Pharmacologic Treatment for Addictions

Clients with an addiction may require pharmacologic interventions. In some cases, when a client has developed a physiological dependence, a medical detoxification may be necessary. Medications to control withdrawal symptoms may be prescribed.

There has been a great deal of controversy about giving clients with an addiction maintenance therapy. For example, heroin addiction is sometimes treated by giving the addict legally prescribed doses of opiates, such as Methadone. The idea behind Methadone maintenance is that the client may have a physiologic need for narcotics that persists despite efforts to withdraw. When addicts are given a legally prescribed supply of the drug, destructive antisocial behaviors, such as theft and violent crime, will decrease. The difficulty with Methadone maintenance is that clients often supplement prescribed doses with illegal street drugs to achieve a desired high.

In addition, Antabuse is sometimes used as a deterrent to discourage alcohol intoxication. Antabuse causes severe nausea when taken with alcohol. Clients addicted to alcohol can voluntarily take this medication as added support for the inhibition of an impulse to drink. If you know you are going to get sick and have to go to the emergency room, you may be less likely to take that first drink. The delay needed to rid the system of Antabuse might provide enough support to wait out a craving. The interaction of Antabuse and alcohol in a person's system can be life-threatening and may required immediate emergency treatment. Clients using this medication should be cautioned about coming into contact with alcohol in hair spray, mouthwash, and skin cleansers, because this interaction also may induce vomiting and a hypertensive crisis.

Narcotic agonists are now being used to prevent clients addicted to narcotics from obtaining the high from these drugs. Agents such as Naltrexone can be prescribed to inhibit the effects of ingested narcotics. This medication is a narcotic agonist and will neutralize the effects of any narcotics absorbed into the person's system. This type of medication was first used in medical/surgical settings to reverse the effects of anesthesia or pain medications. They block the effects of a narcotic so that the person does not get high. Both Antabuse and Naltrexone require that the client voluntarily take the medications. The client must be committed to sobriety and able to comply with a physician's recommendations.

Medications Used for Organic Difficulty

Tegretol is sometimes used to treat abnormal electrical activity in the brain. This medication, traditionally used to treat seizures, has been shown to have positive psychological effects for clients with temporal lobe epilepsy or impulse control disorders. Temporal lobe epilepsy is an impulse disorder that is attributed to abnormal electrical activity. Clients with this condition are prone to emotional outbursts and severe mood swings.

Exciting new discoveries are being made in relation to the treatment of dementia. Several new medications are available to help slow or reverse the effects of organic changes. Cognex has been used for several years with limited success in retarding the dementia process. This medication may need to be taken for up to six months before an effect is noted. As such, it should be tried early on in the dementia process. Another promising new medication, Aricept, has recently been introduced for the treatment of dementia. In its early trials, this medication seems to have a more positive effect for more types of patients, with fewer side effects and reduced liver toxicity.

Combination Therapy

It is not unusual to see combinations of drugs used for treatment. Again, the basic premise is to target specific symptoms with specific agents. However, when used in combination, different agents may potentiate each other's action. That is to say, the drugs will have a synergistic effect when taken together and produce a more powerful effect on symptoms that have not been controlled by a single medication alone. For example, clients with severe mental illness may need an antidepressant used in combination with an antianxiety or antipsychotic agent. A typical combination for someone with chronic mental illness might include Haldol to control hallucinations, Klonopin to potentiate the Haldol and produce reduced anxiety, and Cogentin to control side effects. Someone who is depressed might use Prozac to target depressive symptoms, and Ativan to manage anxiety.

There is an increased risk of side effects when medications are used in combinations. When a client is taking several psychoactive medications they, along with their physician, must be vigilant about monitoring side effects. They need to report any changes, such as blurred vision, constipation, nausea, trembling, ankle swelling, or fatigue. Tell all your physicians what medications you are taking. Use the same pharmacy for filling all your prescriptions so the pharmacist can help keep track of incompatibilities or errors. Make a list of all the medications you use, including over-the-counter preparations, and bring it with you when you visit the physician.

Medications and the Older Adult

As we age, our metabolism slows down. Because of this, elderly clients often require smaller doses of medication. Older adults are at risk for dehydration, particularly when they are struggling with emotional symptoms. Dehydration can also potentiate the effects of medications. Older adults often see several specialists, all prescribing different agents. The different doctors may not even know about each other. Older adults often have developed physical conditions and are taking medications to relieve these symptoms. At times, it is impossible for the client to remember the names of all the different medicines she is taking. Prescriptions might be followed inconsistently or incorrectly. All these factors combine to put the older client at risk for developing serious side effects from medications used to treat psychological disorders. Too many older adults have ended up in the hospital because of overmedication.

This is changing somewhat. Specialists in geropsychiatry and geriatric psychology take special training in working with elderly clients. The older adult body is as different as children are from younger adults. Care givers need specialized training in order to work with these clients. Care providers who work with older adults need to learn how to prescribe specifically for the elder's physical needs, body tolerances, and life-style. Pharmacies are helping by tracking the variety of medications being taken by one person. Pharmacies can also alert clients and physicians when medications are incompatible and should not be given together, or when doses are inappropriate. However, pharmacists will not make recommendations about the clinical condition of the patient and usually do not suggest specific medication changes.

Psychodynamics of Medication

It is impossible to separate the psychological aspects of medications from the biological effects. Because prescribing always takes place within a human system and within a relationship, understanding the dynamics of medication is an essential part of treatment. The meaning of the exchange of a medication, both conscious and unconscious, may impact how well the medication works. If a client believes that medication will be helpful, they may be more likely to be aware of positive effects and minimize the perception of side effects.

Clinicians offer medications with a genuine desire to help alleviate symptoms. As such, suggesting a prescription can be viewed as an act of giving or caring. Often, a clinician is moved to offer medications because the suffering caused by symptoms is hard to bear—for the client and therapist alike. Clinicians need to consider carefully why they might be offering medications at a specific point in therapy. Is it clinically indicated to suppress symptoms rather than experience and tolerate them? If the answer is yes, then it is appropriate to use medications. If it is advisable to minimize distress and to suppress symptoms, the use of medications may be indicated. However, if it might be more useful to bear the emotions and successfully work through a resolution to the distress, medications might inhibit progress in treatment.

Some clients may be reluctant to take medications because of conflicts about dependency issues. Some clients fear developing a physiological addiction, and with some medications this is a valid concern. Others report that they don't want to rely on medicine "for the rest of my life." At some level, they see needing a medication as evidence of some inner defect or central failing. It is as if admitting that there is a biological neurotransmitter imbalance is acknowledgment of some core, shameful defect. For some people it is hard to view diminished levels of serotonin in depression with the same nonjudgment that we view diminished levels of insulin in diabetes.

Medications taken orally are literally ingested by the client. In a primitive, unconscious way, this may symbolically represent ingesting the therapist. The effects of the therapist are literally inside the person. The therapist is incorporated into the client's actual physical being, and wishes of oral dependence may be satisfied. By taking a medicine that is prescribed by the therapist, it is as if he is with the client always, supporting well-being internally and literally. Clients sometimes demand medications because they need to feel supported and cared about by the therapist.

If a client is reluctant to take medications, the recommendation of a prescription might feel like an intrusion from the therapist. If a physician orders injectable medication, the client may feel particularly assaulted by the therapist. If medications have unpleasant side effects, the client may unconsciously feel the therapist is responsible.

Because of these relationship issues, some therapists prefer to separate the duties of prescribing from the process of psychotherapy. Consultations with different clinicians can be arranged to accommodate the client's needs. These clinicians may collaborate about the progress of the client while maintaining different goals for therapeutic work.

Pharmacotherapy is generally most effective when combined with psychotherapy. Studies on the treatment of depression have shown that the combination of antidepressants and therapy was more effective than either treatment alone, or placebo groups. Medications can help to alleviate severe symptoms and make the work of psychotherapy possible.

Other Biological Treatments

There have been many attempts to alleviate symptoms through a biological approach. In retrospect, the history of biological interventions may seem at once comical and alarming. It is important to keep in mind that clinicians who developed these interventions were well-meaning and attempting to be therapeutic. They were constrained by the limitations of scientific knowledge of their day.

Some of the most primitive attempts to alter behavior are found in ancient civilizations. Trephining was a common practice designed to release evil spirits from the personality and brain. Trephining involves placing a burr hole in someone's skull, with the intention of allowing unwanted influences to escape.

Ancient medicine traced psychological difficulties to imbalances in the body's fluids, or humors. They believed that optimal adjustment was the result of a balance between black bile, yellow bile, blood, and phlegm. For example, someone who was easygoing, perhaps even lazy, was said to have an excess of blood, giving rise to a sanguine personality.

One of the earliest modern biophysical interventions was phrenology, the science of understanding personality through the bumps on the scalp, and producing symptom relief through pressure on selected regions of the skull. Even Freud's early treatments involved pressing on the head to evoke memories that would be useful. Metal helmets designed to apply pressure to selected areas of the skull were fashioned and applied for specified periods of time.

Behavioral change was noted to occur in clients who experienced insulin shock as a result of a disease process. This led to attempts to induce a temporary coma with insulin therapy in those with chronic mental illness that had not responded to conventional treatment.

Perhaps the most well-known and controversial biological treatment is the lobotomy. It was noted that when a client experienced physical destruction of parts of the brain, a more docile personality was often the result. Attempts to produce behavioral change by destroying parts of the frontal lobe appeared to have some success. However, results of this nonspecific damage often left a client with unintended cognitive impairments.

Electroconvulsive Treatment

Many people are surprised to find out that shock therapy is still used today. I was horrified the first time I assisted in the administration of electroconvulsive therapy (ECT). In an earlier paper in college, I had researched and presented arguments to ban the use of this type of treatment and believed it to be alarmingly inhumane. Through the course of my work at a university hospital, I helped to take care of a young woman who was experiencing severe depression that had left her with altered perceptions of reality. Her depression had progressed so far that she was hearing voices telling her to kill herself. She had come into the hospital after making a serious attempt to take her own life. I was alarmed when her treating psychiatrists suggested ECT. I was ignorant about the potential benefits of this type of treatment and misinformed about the procedure and its potential side effects.

Her psychiatrists were concerned about waiting for antidepressant medication to take effect. Agents available to treat depression at that time often took several weeks to make any positive changes. While waiting for those changes, this client was at risk of harming herself again. The clinicians were aware that ECT might offer some immediate relief that would make tolerable the wait for relief from medications.

I was assigned to accompany this client for her first treatment. I was delighted to discover that with the assistance of anesthesia, the procedure was uneventful, even routine. The client tolerated the procedure without any side effects and began to feel relief from her depression after only two treatments.

There have been vocal opponents of the use of shock therapy, as well as a history of controversy surrounding the procedure. However, electroconvulsive therapy may be the treatment of choice for some individuals with depression. Often, the relief obtained after one or two treatments can be remarkable. Objections to shock therapy can be traced back to the days when it was widely used on institutionalized clients with chronic mental illness. Legitimate concerns about inpatient client's rights prompted restrictions on the use of ECT.

Practicing clinicians noted that seizures had an important effect on mood and behavior in epileptic clients. Psychiatrists began to induce seizures in clients by using electric energy applied to strategic brain regions. Results showed dramatic improvement in depression, as well as psychotic symptoms. In its early forms, ECT did not use any anesthesia, so the client was painfully aware of the shock itself. The seizure activity also resulted in tonic movements that often resulted in fractures of the bones in the arms and legs.

Today, electroconvulsive treatment is done using general anesthesia and is a pain-free procedure. The client is given an antianxiety agent that decreases awareness of the procedure. In addition, clients are given muscle-relaxing agents that prevent the classic movements associated with a grand mal seizure. Low voltages of current are used to minimize side effects but achieve maximal therapeutic effect. Clinicians have learned that if electrodes are placed only on one side of the brain, temporary impairment of memory is minimized.

Electroconvulsive treatment may be indicated for clients who are elderly and who might not be able to tolerate the adverse effects of medications. Many antidepressants have cardiac side effects and cannot be used by an elderly client with a heart condition. Depression that has not responded to medications may respond to ECT.

ECT is generally contraindicated if a client has previous

brain damage or organic impairment. Clients need to be physically strong enough to tolerate a brief period of sedation and the effects of anesthesia. Clients with brittle bones or osteoporosis may not be candidates for the procedure.

ECT can have important psychological implications. When a clinician recommends ECT in the context of a psychotherapy, there may be a significant impact on the treatment relationship. Clients may have misconceptions about ECT and fear the treatment. If ECT is recommended, clients may view themselves as failing at other forms of treatment.

It is unusual for a client to request ECT spontaneously. When a client is asking for shock therapy, the motivations for this request must be thoroughly understood. A client who is preoccupied with self-abuse or self-punishment may seek ECT as a way to enact these fantasies with the psychotherapist. It is a good idea to separate consultation after ECT from any ongoing psychotherapy. A separate clinician should evaluate the need for and administer the treatment if necessary.

Psychosurgery

Physical alterations to brain structure have been attempted as a means of alleviating severe mental illness. To help clients with severe behavioral difficulties, surgical techniques that were designed to quiet brain activity were developed. During the 1950s this treatment was widely used. The prefrontal lobotomy was used more than thirty thousand times in the United States prior to the invention of Thorazine. Although in retrospect this intervention seems cruel, keep in mind that clinicians had intentions of helping when they applied this form of treatment. Lobotomies were applied to patients with severe agitation, unremitting hallucinations, and violent acting out. The rationale for the treatment was that the behavior would be interrupted if the brain tissue that supported it was destroyed. In its earliest form, the lobotomy was nonspecific about the areas that were ablated (or destroyed). Clinicians found that clients who had part of the frontal lobe destroyed had an increase in docile behavior, and their thinking was less disturbed. As physicians learned more about brain structure and function, this practice was all but abandoned. However, surgical techniques for alleviating mental distress are under investigation and are used in extreme cases with a clear biological origin. For example, if a client is having seizures that disrupt behavior, the area of the brain involved in the seizure may be ablated, so impulses are rerouted and seizures are interrupted. Using today's techniques, any surgical interruption of brain structure is microscopic. Microscopic areas of the brain are also altered now that we have increased knowledge of the functional aspects of brain tissue.

Psychoneuroimmunology (PNI)

PNI is the science of how the mind influences neurological and immune-system responses. We have observed that stress has an impact on our psychological, neurological, and immune systems. How these three systems interact and respond to stresses in the environment is the subject of a significant amount of current research. Mental state has a significant impact on physical states of well-being. There seems to be a connection between actual coping abilities, positive mental state, and physical wellness.

We have learned that cells in the brain, endocrine, and immune systems produce chemical messengers called neuropeptides, the chemical link between the mind and the body. These messengers are made during times of positive mental states. This pathway between mind and body can be used to influence well-being.

Deepak Chopra, M.D., a nationally noted physician, author, and public speaker, who combines Ayurveda methods with Western medicine, suggests that cells have a wisdom about self-repair and self-development. He supports the belief that the body is constantly responding to information received from the environment. Awareness of states of stress creates a predictable set of responses, down to a cellular level. If we are able to influence our experiences of stress, we can also alter our body's patterns of physical responding. Of course, we know this because we can see the body react to states of mind simply by observing patterns of breathing. Meditators have known for centuries that mental state influences physical well-being. In 1992, the National Institutes of Health formed the Office of Alternative Medicine (OAM) to study the effects of alternative therapies. The OAM is actively investigating how stress and the immune system interact and which methods are most effective in reducing stress.

Genetic Research

Currently, medical and biological scientists are in a race to map human DNA. (DNA and RNA are the messengers that carry our genetic code to our cells as they develop and reproduce.) The information contained in these messengers determine to a significant degree our physical, mental, and emotional characteristics. Some theorists suggest that there is a genetic basis for many mental illnesses. There is strong evidence to support this view. In many disorders, twins with the same DNA are significantly more likely to develop certain psychological illnesses than people with different genetic material. For certain disorders, a family history significantly increases the chances that a person will develop the same condition. The strongest evidence for a genetic underpinning is found in the schizophrenias, some degenerative neurologic disorders, and some mood disorders. We are still not sure exactly how much of who we are is related to genes and how much to other factors. We cannot explain why two people who possess the same genetic tendencies will express different manifest characteristics. Although clinicians have debated about how much of a role genetics can play, there is no doubt that genes do have an impact on mental health.

Scientists hope to be able to identify specific genes related to specific disorders. This is a painstaking and arduous task. If it becomes possible for us to identify specific genetic markers, we might be able to develop interventions to counteract these effects. Education about genetic tendencies can assist individuals in making choices about having children. Treatment using gene therapy is in the early phases of preliminary investigation, and it may be years before these theories have an applied role in the clinical setting.

CHAPTER 9

Children and Therapy

C hildhood is not an easy time. Anyone who says, "I had a happy childhood" is either unusually lucky, or they are using some measure of repression. Childhood is a time of enormous developmental challenge. Children are in perpetual biological flux, as growth and development occur at a rapid rate. In functional families, adults in the environment provide what the child needs in order to meet developmental challenges and feel satisfied and secure. However, in some families adults have unmet needs, and as they work on meeting their own adult needs, the child's concerns can go unaddressed. The child automatically and unconsciously begins to help the adults in their world to get their needs met. In so doing, the child increases the likelihood that their own concerns will be addressed. In dysfunctional families, children provide care for their parents because to *not* do so is to risk their own survival. The parents must survive in order to take care of the children, and the children know and respond to this. Ideally, parents should be supported enough in their environment to be available to concentrate on providing for the needs of the children until they are able to provide for themselves.

A child does not exist in a vacuum. Children tend to develop problems in response to environmental systems. Generally, a child does not come to therapy alone. Treatment must work with the members of the child's system and involve care givers. Even if a child is living away from the family—in residential treatment, for example—the child's behavior is often an expression of a reaction to the environment. It is essential that a child's behavioral difficulties be understood within the context of the care-providing system.

Children express themselves symbolically through behaviors, including play. The imagination is a projective. For the child, all activity is expression. In children, we accept that there will be a wide variation in behavioral expression across an age range. Imagination and emotions are expected to be vivid and dramatic. There is a much wider variation in the behavior tolerated in children compared with what is tolerated in adults. When a child presents with a behavior or characteristic that is problematic, we must first consider developmental norms. What are the expected behaviors of this age? What are the normal developmental challenges that a child of this age is addressing? Is behavior age-appropriate, or do elements of the behavior belong to a characteristically younger or older age?

Family Functioning

It seems as if the functional family is an urban myth perpetuated by television shows such as "The Brady Bunch," "The Dick Van Dyke Show," and "The Waltons." Dysfunction appears to be the norm, and families that appear normal are really just better at hiding their dirty laundry from the view of curious onlookers. Ideally, the family is a place that supports our sense of security. A healthy family fosters self-acceptance and validation of our views of the world. Ideally, in our families we feel loved and accepted. Home is ideally a place where we can be ourselves and know that it is alright. A functional family provides an environment that supports and encourages personal development. Families can provide for refueling, as well as replenish energy to fight the battles of the world. It is only in recent history that people marry for love. In the past, economic necessity was often the foundation for sustaining marriage and family. In an agrarian society, children represented potential economic resources.

Functional families respect privacy and have consistent boundaries between subgroups. Parents share common time and information. Children are viewed as separate individuals. Ideal family communication allows for the expression of all points of view, with an ultimate structure coming from parents with consistent and sensitive styles. The family functions as a system, drawing from available resources and solving problems with a group mentality. Family loyalty is often fostered by mutual dependence on family members.

The reality of family relationships is both positive and negative. Individuals bring to their family relationships limitations in personal functioning. For example, if parents are highly focused on their own unmet needs, they will likely neglect the needs of their children. Family structure is significantly influenced by our families of origin. From our early family experiences, we learn what a family is and how it supposedly functions. We watch our parents relate to each other and to us. We form opinions about what family is and how people are expected to relate. Difficulties arise when parents provide less than ideal role models for family patterns.

Modern culture allows the commitment of marriage to be more easily dissolved, and divorce is a common occurrence. The contemporary family hardly resembles the nuclear group of the 1950s: mom, dad, and three kids. Today it is much more common to find remarriages and children from different biological parents living together in combined households.

Grandparents frequently raise the children, as parents are forced to work outside the home.

When family boundaries are too fluid or too rigid, children may be injured in damaging interactions. An example of a too fluid boundary is in physical or sexual abuse. Here, the child's right to be free from exploitation is ignored, and the child is used for the purpose of meeting the adult's needs. This can happen through too much love and closeness. If a parent has too much need for admiration, devotion, and love from the child, they may not be able to respect the child's needs for autonomy. The parent may expect the child to be around for the purpose of providing emotional nurturance. The child is not free to live her own life, as she has a job from a very early age. An example of boundaries that are too rigid may involve expectations that are too high for the child. The parent may need the child to excel at sports, for example, or school. Punishments for failure may be severe.

Family therapy is generally not covered by third-party reimbursement. It is difficult to say how much time was spent on each individual, therefore it is difficult to identify a client. Insurance companies rely on the difficulty of identifying who the client is, and exactly how he was treated as a rationale for not covering family therapy. An exception is made for collateral family visits. In this case, one family member is identified as the primary patient. Often, this is a child with behavioral or school difficulties. Some insurance plans will reimburse for sessions that involve family members where the focus is on resolving the difficulties of the primary client.

When Should a Child Have Therapy?

Knowing when a child should have counseling is sometimes difficult to determine. This is because a wide range of behaviors and feelings can occur as a result of normal variations in development. We tolerate a much wider range of actions and fluctuations in functioning in children. Adaptation during childhood is much more fluid that in adulthood. Abilities change and mastery of new challenges is an evolving process in children. Young children are learning to master their emotions, so outbursts and lively expressions are to be expected.

Whenever you wonder about whether a child's behavior is symptomatic, you must first ask yourself, "What are expected behavioral norms for the child's developmental level?" Behaviors can only be evaluated in a developmental context. Keep in mind that normal progression through the phases of growing produces conflicts and challenges to adaptive capacities. Parents can be supported in dealing with these maturational crises, but care should be taken not to label these behaviors as pathologic or abnormal.

Children who are not yet school-age should see a therapist if there is a significant lag in achieving developmental milestones. A complete physical examination by a pediatrician should be performed to make sure that there are no underlying illnesses or diseases. For example, if a child is significantly slower than most to talk, and consultation with a pediatrician reveals no physical abnormalities, an assessment by a therapist might be indicated. A therapist can evaluate the child's needs and assess how family resources can be arranged to effectively address these needs.

The best indicators of difficulty in children may be their school functioning. Behavior that may have been adapted to or tolerated within the family is recognized as inappropriate when the child enters a school setting. School is a child's work. When an adult has emotional difficulties, it is often apparent in his work performance. The same is true of children. Children may have difficulty socializing with peers or accomplishing intellectual tasks. School requires that a child develop impulse-control skills and manners to interact appropriately with adults and peers. Take particular notice if a child who has previously been doing well develops sudden difficulties. A sudden drop in adjustment may indicate family or interpersonal stresses.

Families that are at risk such as teen parents, might seek preventive counseling and assistance in developing parenting skills when a child is still in infancy. When counseling services are used early in a family's development, later disorders can be avoided.

Parental Perceptions

Parents' attitudes about children and psychotherapy have an impact on decisions about seeking treatment. From the moment a child is planned, parents have expectations. Parents may feel mortified when their children have behavioral difficulties. There can be a sense of shame at having failed at that most sacred of duties—raising children. Feeling that "I'm a bad mom" or "I'm not a good dad," may surface when parents think about therapy for their children.

One parental attitude is particularly disturbing. I have heard parents threaten children, especially teenagers, with therapy. Therapy is used as a punishment or a way of making a child feel crazy or abnormal. Parents may be tempted to say, "If your grades don't improve, I'm taking you to a therapist." This sets up therapy as a negative consequence. It may be more effective for parents to sketch the therapy process as a consultation for support and an opportunity to learn new perspectives and problem-solving methods.

Parents sometimes expect to drop children off at a therapist to have them fixed. This is also unrealistic. Parents can expect to participate actively in most types of therapy that involve children. Children cannot be *fixed*; they are influenced. Parents need to be aware of what is happening in therapy and be able to support the work at home.

Consent with Children

A major difference in therapy with children is that they are generally brought for treatment by their parents. Frequently, there are difficult feelings between the parent and child. If the child is at an age where she is asserting autonomy, this may be displayed by resisting actively engaging in therapy. However, most children quickly become involved and enjoy the therapist's attention and concentration. If a child persists in refusing to participate in treatment, some other form, such as family therapy, may be indicated.

Children have some special considerations in the eyes of the law in relation to consent for treatment. For a child to enter into outpatient therapy, he must have the consent of his parent or guardian. One exception is the right to enter into treatment for drug and alcohol problems without informing parents. However, the law stipulates that a child has the right to seek inpatient treatment after the age of fourteen, with his own consent. The hospital has a duty to inform the parents of the child's whereabouts but does not need their permission if the child is requesting treatment. These statutes recognize that during adolescence, such mental struggles may arise, and that the teen has gained autonomy to request evaluation and help, even when the parents disagree. A hearing will be held subsequent to the initiation of treatment in order to assess the best interests of the child.

Play Therapy

Children have a natural tendency to express themselves in action because their ability to verbally articulate concerns is limited depending on their age. It is normal for children to express themselves through activity or, more commonly, play. As a result, when young children enter into therapy, the medium of communication is often play. It is important for parents to realize that play is meaningful and that it can be understood in much the same way that dreams can be understood.

Understanding what is happening in play therapy is difficult at best. I have often found that working with children involves inherent confusion. As a therapist, I remain interested and diligent about trying to understand communications and symbolism, but often, the child's meaning cannot be fully appreciated. When a child plays in therapy, they are communicating whatever issues are most important. Often, child's play is carried on without drawing much attention from adults. However, by observing play, it is possible to view the child's mental functioning. Even when a child appears to be uninvolved in treatment, behaviors and expressions are never casual or idle. Every motion contains a communication. Luckily, children are tenacious. They will communicate the same message repeatedly until adults in the environment attend to it.

Once a mother brought her son to sessions because she had concerns about his adjustment to a recent divorce. The child was only five and was conspicuously silent during our first session. The mother repeatedly encouraged him to talk to the *nice therapist,* but the child answered questions with soft, one-word answers. However, while the mother and therapist were discussing current concerns, the child began to tentatively manipulate toys in the therapy room. He appeared uninterested in the therapist's conversation and ignored the adults as he began to draw. When the therapist announced that there were only ten minutes remaining in the session, the child silently took out two playhouses. He separated the houses, placed a mommy doll in one house, and a daddy doll in the other. He then placed a third doll in a school bus and drove it repeatedly back and forth between the two houses. Had the therapist insisted that the child talk, instead of allowing him to evolve his own unique expression, the child might have been overwhelmed by the process. Clearly, he was playing out the essential conflict for the therapist to observe. Learning to monitor a child's mental activity by observing his play can be extremely helpful in assisting the child to master current conflicts.

Children in therapy have a broad range of expressions. One adolescent client played the guitar for a therapist when they were unable to process information verbally. Some children draw. Some play, while others do all their work in conversation. For children, therapy presents a unique relationship with an adult. Receiving sustained attention at regular intervals is, sadly, a rare occurrence for many children. When I work with children, I have only two rules in-session: Nobody gets hurt, and nothing gets broken. Most children are able to conduct themselves in accordance with these rules. The nobody gets hurt rule might need to be invoked when a child is very physical in-session. Feedback such as "that hurts" is a reality check. Nothing gets broken extends to include any damage to property. So, for example, if a child is in danger of damaging wood furniture with Play-Doh, the therapist needs to support the child in staying within the rules. A mat can be obtained to protect both the child and the furniture.

Adolescents

It seems that along with the hormonal turmoil that accompanies puberty, so should a referral to a counselor. Every teenager ought to have a protected right to see a therapist. It is a confusing time of defining the self, of testing limits and boundaries, of exploring sexuality and identity. Even a normal adolescent can benefit from talking things over with a trusted counselor. However, most teens see counselors as being on the *adult* team, not as someone to be confided in. In addition, it is usually the parent who insists on therapy, often threatening the teen, saying, "If your behavior doesn't improve, you're going to counseling!" When placed in this punishing context, it is not hard to see why teenagers often come to therapy reluctantly. In addition, teens strive most to be like their peers. They want to belong to the crowd, not stand out as individuals. If they admit that something is wrong, or they have some problems they cannot manage, they are admitting, "I am different," something a teen is averse to doing. It is also a blow to newfound autonomy to have to ask for help. These factors often make it difficult for a teen to form an alliance with a therapist.

However, if a therapist can gradually earn the teen client's trust and respect, a beneficial alliance can be formed. On the other hand, some teens take readily to the therapy process. They can be relieved at having someone on their side, and feel less anxious knowing the counselor will help with problem solving. When a teen is concerned about serious symptoms, they are sometimes eager to discuss them with a therapist. The teen can use the therapy to affirm a developing identity. The relationship can serve as a setting for exploring choices that come with increasing freedom and responsibility. Often, a teen feels as if no one understands them. The therapist can give the teen an opportunity to experience diligent, sustained attention that is devoted to understanding their existence.

College Counseling Centers

Late adolescence is a challenging era and may involve leaving home, beginning work, or attending college. Most colleges make some provisions for offering counseling to students. Often, an evaluation and several sessions may be free of charge. Some schools have counseling departments that offer comprehensive services. Others may refer to local therapists who specialize in young-adult clients.

Seeking treatment at a college counseling center is a good

idea because it is easily accessible. If the counseling center is active on campus, the stigma of asking for guidance or support may be reduced. Counselors who understand the unique challenges of this developmental time and the climate of the campus life may be better able to communicate with these clients. In addition, the young adult can access these services independently, without the involvement of parents. They may feel more inclined to use the work of therapy effectively rather than being resistant to being brought to a therapist chosen by their parents.

Counseling centers can be helpful in addressing issues of time management and stress reduction, as well as addressing developmental challenges and relationship difficulties. Most counseling centers are not set up to manage severe chronic illness. When symptoms are severe and more extensive services are needed, a college-based center may refer to local and community resources for the student.

Disorders First Evident During Childhood

Childhood is not an easy time. Many children will show some evidence of symptoms at some point during development. Symptoms may be related to developmental challenges, genetic or biological variations, or situational stresses. Because such a wide range of behavior is accepted in chidden, generally, when a child comes to the attention of a professional therapist, symptoms are relatively serious.

Learning Disabilities

School difficulties are the impetus for consultation for many children. When a child achieves at a rate that is significantly slower than expected norms, a learning disability may be suspected. There are many types of learning difficulties: difficulty with auditory or visual processing; specific skill disorders; or global impairment in learning processes. Generally, when a diagnosis of learning disability is made, no significant neurological impairments are found. These children have *soft signs* of biological involvement. Diffuse difficulties with cognitive processing are common. Psychologists are skilled at assessing functional deficits in order to develop a plan of remediation.

Mental Retardation

Mental retardation involves both intellectual and social deficits. It can be caused by alterations in chromosomes, biological insult, nutritional complications, or environmental deprivation. Clients with mild retardation are able to work in a supported environment and can master many of the skills of daily living. Moderate retardation may impair self-care abilities, and vocational activities will require supervision. Clients with severe retardation will need assistance with activities of daily living and almost continuous supervision. Clients with profound retardation may not be able to communicate and will need assistance with physical needs.

Depression

As we recall childhood with rose-colored glasses, it may be difficult to comprehend that children sometimes become depressed. Depression in children is somewhat common, as they react to losses that are inherent in development. Even infants will exhibit depression when care giving is inadequate. Children have easy access to their emotions, and from an early age can identify feelings of sadness, hopelessness, anger, and fear. Fortunately, for most children these emotions are transient and short-lived.

Depression in children is often similar to what is seen in

depressed adults. The child may say they are depressed, blue, or sad. Disinterest in activities that the child previously enjoyed may be evident. He may have changes in sleep patterns, appetite, or energy levels, and might feel guilty or have low self-esteem. Children do think about suicide at times. Parents may notice an increase in risky behaviors because the child has become unconcerned about his own death. Accidents should be investigated fully to assess for hidden impulses to self-harm.

Autism

Symptoms of autism are generally apparent in a child before the age of two and a half. The child may exhibit difficulty with relationships and prefer to attend to inner stimuli rather than interacting with care givers. There may be ritualistic behaviors or rhythmic movements, such as rocking. The child's attention appears to become focused on details that he studies for hours. Language fails to develop normally. There may be episodes of extreme excitability when the child becomes overwhelmed with stimuli.

The causes of autism are poorly understood. We suspect that there is a biological or neurological deficit that accounts for the aberrations in behavior, but research has not been able to identify a specific mechanism. Treatment for autism generally involves altering the environmental stimuli to support adaptive behavior, which may include limiting stimuli and rewarding desired behavior.

Anxiety Disorders

Separation anxiety is a universal experience in childhood. There are two normal peaks in this type of anxiety: at nine months and about three years. At nine months, children normally go through a period of increased anxiety at the recognition of strangers. When the infant encounters a person who is unfamiliar, she may utter fearful screams. A recurrence of anxiety is expected during the rapprochement phase of separation-individuation. As the child negotiates her autonomy from parents, her realization of separation gives rise to panic. These experiences are all in the range of normal development. When a child is successful in negotiating these challenges, future separations are likely to be less eventful.

It can be common for children to develop anxiety disorders when they attend school. A child may even refuse to go despite the parent's insistence. The child may exhibit tantrums that are characteristic of a younger age.

Attention Deficit Disorder

The disorder of the 1990s seems to be Attention Deficit Disorder (ADD). Many children come to the attention of a therapist because of difficulties in school. These difficulties may involve inability to concentrate on tasks or fidgety behavior during class. The diagnosis of ADD or Attention Deficit Hyperactivity Disorder (ADHD) should not be given without a thorough examination of the child, the setting, and the behavior. Alterations in the child's environment or patterns of care should be attempted before medications are tried. The times when ADD or ADHD will require Ritalin are rare.

The Psychotic Child

Children, by nature, spend a great deal of time in fantasy. A child's thinking is not governed by the rules of logical adult thought. However, at times a child may break from reality in a way that is more than just imagination. Like adults, children can experience hallucinations and delusions. For example a child might begin to believe his food is poisoned. He might even stop eating because of this belief. No amount of evidence can convince him otherwise. This is a delusion. Hallucinations may be more difficult to assess because children have vivid imaginations and frequently see images we don't. Children also commonly will play with imaginary friends, who are considered normal until an age when thinking becomes more realistic.

The difference between imagination and hallucinations is essentially voluntary control. With some effort, the child is able to refocus thinking when imagination is at play. An hallucination is not under voluntary, conscious control.

When a child fails to develop normal contact with reality from earliest life, a diagnosis of autism is generally applied. Autism involves a failure to develop patterns of interaction with significant others. The child remains preoccupied with an inner reality. If a child develops normally but begins to experience symptoms of internal preoccupation and behavioral withdrawal, a diagnosis of childhood schizophrenia may be applied.

The psychotic child may be helped by a consistent, firm but loving environment. Care givers may need to alter environmental stimuli to match the capabilities of the child's psyche. If given in small doses, medications may be helpful.

Personality Disorders

Children may have alterations in their character development. A child may develop an oppositional disposition and refuse to take directions from adults. The child with oppositional defiant disorder will have frequent arguments with adults. Conduct disorder involves behavioral symptoms that include destruction of property and a disregard for the rights of humans or animals.

Testing for Children

Most children encounter some form of developmental testing as a part of formal school evaluations. Teachers and schools are set up to screen for children with cognitive or intellectual difficulties. Every school district has a psychologist to provide evaluation and treatment of children who are identified as at risk or having recognized impairments. If a child is performing outside the range of expected norms, an evaluation of intellectual capacity may be recommended by the school district.

Intellectual functioning is assessed using either the Stanford Binet, or the Weschler Intelligence Test for Children, now in its third edition. If there is a suggestion of personality or emotional difficulty, projective instruments may be added to the test battery. These include the Child Apperception Test and the Rorscharch inkblot tests. Psychologists can use these instruments to assess areas of strength and limitation, as well as design a program that will optimize functioning and adjustment.

Inpatient Treatment for Children

Children are rarely removed from their families for treatment. Today, in-home services can be provided with skilled support staff. Known as wraparound services, they can implement family and behavioral treatment in the child's own environment. Coordination of services between school and home environments is accomplished by a team leader who fashions an individualized treatment plan.

However, there may be times when intervention from an inpatient setting can be helpful. Children are hospitalized when their care givers become exhausted, and resources for meeting the child's needs are overwhelmed. Brief periods of hospitalization may allow for evaluation of problem behaviors and emotions.

Wraparound Services

Rather than removing children from their living environment, these days the trend is to use in-home support services to assist the child and the family with coping. These services carry the benefits of a cost savings over institutionalization and for helping the family unit to stay intact. The child is assisted to achieve desired goals within the context of the family. Wraparound services involve a treatment team that comes to the home and works with the child and the family. Generally, a professional therapist assesses the difficulty and develops a treatment plan in consultation with the child and the primary care givers. Services may include support staff members who can provide supplemental care in the home setting. A counselor might stay with the child for several hours, or around-the-clock coverage can be arranged for clients with severe difficulties. These counselors can provide ongoing behavioral support and assist with implementing prescribed treatment approaches.

Using Medications with Children

Medications in children should be used with extreme caution. Most often, symptomatic behavior in children is a result of some dysfunction in the family system. Giving a child medication without considering the origin of the symptoms is irresponsible. When we encourage children to cope with symptoms by using medications, we may be establishing a life-long pattern that promotes the use of drugs. Parents must be taught how to help the child to gain mobile cognitive and emotional resources, and reserve the use of medications for only the most extreme situations.

Antidepressants

Antidepressants may have some limited use with children who have severe symptoms of depression. Children do get severely depressed. We have a collective adult fantasy that childhood is a time of innocence and happiness. The reality is that childhood is an arduous time of few personal rights and even fewer freedoms. Children frequently feel lonely, ashamed, or incompetent by virtue of the normal developmental tasks. When life presents extraordinary loss or injuries, children will become clinically depressed. In addition to beginning a talking therapy, small doses of traditional antidepressants may be useful. Doses are age- and size-dependent and should be titrated to reduce any side effects.

Ritalin

Ritalin has undoubtedly been overprescribed. It is a stimulant that has shown to be beneficial in reducing behavioral symptoms associated with hyperactivity. In essence, ADD and ADHD can be understood as understimulation of the child's brain activity. By ingesting a stimulant, the mental functioning is brought in line with current levels of thought processing. Parents who are frustrated by their child's behavioral difficulties frequently seek consultation and suspect a diagnosis of ADD/ADHD. They ask for Ritalin because they have heard stories about its beneficial effects. Unfortunately, clinicians have been too broad in their interpretations of the indications for Ritalin prescription. Before it is prescribed, changes in the child's environment and schedule should be implemented. It is true that a child who is bored will often become fidgety, restless, irritable, and contrary. Increasing the structure and the stimulus for these children is preferable to medicating them.

Antipsychotics

For the small percentage of children that has impaired reality testing, there may be a role for antipsychotic medications. Again, the environment should be altered before medications are tried, and increased structure should be put in place to attempt to reduce symptoms. Antipsychotic medications can be used in small doses to help the child organize thoughts.

CHAPTER 10

Additional Forms of Therapy

Crisis Intervention

There may be times in life when psychological and emotional difficulties reach a point of crisis. Anyone can be overwhelmed by a sudden traumatic event or circumstance. Crisis intervention assumes that the client is basically healthy and that the presenting problem is a time-limited, normal response to overwhelming circumstances. Crisis intervention is appropriate when the presenting difficulty is not symptomatic of some underlying psychological difficulty.

The focus of crisis intervention is finding a resolution for the immediate problem. It is directed at present issues, not the past. Treatment recommendations may include small changes, with a belief that accomplishing short-term goals will increase the likelihood of achieving permanent change. The goal of crisis intervention is to support the client's existing coping mechanisms, as well as restore functioning to precrisis levels.

Brief Psychotherapy

Recently, a new form of therapy has become popular. Called brief psychotherapy, it is a response to the demand for effective, short-term interventions. Because of pressures of cost containment, this new form of therapy is being used with increasing frequency. Brief psychotherapy may involve as little as a single session or as many as twenty. Brief psychotherapy has specific, limited goals. Used appropriately, it is a useful technique for relieving distress.

Brief psychotherapy uses psychodynamic theory as an underlying framework. It is different from crisis intervention in that therapists who do brief therapy are more likely to be clinically trained professionals. Crisis-intervention workers are often trained specifically to deal with crises. It assumes no underlying problems. However, brief pychotherapy assumes that the client has some underlying psychopathology influencing current difficulties. Techniques include addressing specific issues, focusing on the past, and understanding the unconscious. Brief therapy focuses on resolving maladaptive symptoms. It includes an analysis of the past and an understanding of the effect of the past on the present. An added focus in brief psychotherapy is identifying the unconscious processes underlying the difficulty. However, working through issues is left to the client. Although transference may begin to develop, efforts to avoid an intense transference reaction are made by the therapist. Working through a full transference neurosis requires a longer duration of treatment than brief psychotherapy can allow.

Self-Help

Perhaps we would not need to seek professional help so often if only we listened to ourselves more closely. For some people, self-help is an attractive option. Indeed, many of life's problems can be overcome with support and information, and self-healing abilities.

When a group of people without any special training comes together for support or to work on common issues, it is called self-help. Self-help groups do not require a skilled therapist in order to function. Participants rely on the resources available from the members of the group in mastering challenges. One of the largest self-help groups is the National Alliance for the Mentally Ill (NAMI), which comprises clients with mental illness, and their families. This group organizes supportive meetings and educational events, and sponsors legislative change. Other examples of self-help groups include Compassionate Friends, an active organization that provides a support group for parents who have lost children.

Self-help is different from psychotherapy in several ways. It does not involve a skilled care giver. The client is using her own resources to decide what will most benefit the problematic situation. This self-reliance is often the optimal choice for coping, as long as desired results can be achieved. Self-help methods are not individually developed or tailored specifically to your needs. The program is offered as is, and the client bears the responsibility for tailoring support to meet individual needs. For example, a computer program designed to screen for certain diagnostic categories cannot interpret individual nuances and personality. A book with advice on coping is designed to reach a mass audience.

Support groups involve people with common interests or experiences. They may help you feel less alone and isolated. Individuals who share common experiences benefit from a sense of camaraderie as they explore their personal distress. Support groups allow for friendships to develop. These relationships are established in a setting that acknowledges issues and difficulties that might be hidden in other interpersonal settings. For example, if a client worries that intimate relationships will reveal previous experiences with addictive difficulties, relationships established at an addiction support group incorporate these issues into ordinary interactions. People who meet at grief-recovery support groups may feel more free to discuss feelings of loss, when others are uncomfortable with these discussions. Feelings of shame or fears of discovery can be mitigated because participants with similar experiences are less likely to respond judgmentally.

Support groups can offer important breaking news about illness and options for recovery. Networking through national organizations or the Internet can help you stay informed about the latest resources, information, and research on particular disorders.

Self-help groups generally have an open-membership policy, and anyone with an interest is encouraged to attend meetings. Members will be at different levels of recovery, some farther along than others. Members who have attained some resolution of difficulties can pass along what they have learned to those in earlier stages of recovery.

Twelve-Step Fellowship

Twelve-step fellowship is an amazing phenomenon. It has helped countless numbers of people to achieve sobriety and release from addiction. It is absolutely free. It is international. Clients struggling with addiction can find support in their peers, day or night, in any country in the world. Although Alcoholics Anonymous is the largest and most successful of the twelve-step fellowships, narcotics, cocaine, gambling, overeating, shopping, and sex addiction are also addressed in twelve-step groups.

During Prohibition, alcohol use began to rise, and as a result, dependence on alcohol became an increasing problem. Mainstream medical and psychological practitioners were often frustrated by the tenacity of alcohol problems. Clients with alcohol addiction refused to follow their health instructions and continued drinking despite their doctors' best efforts. Psychotherapy didn't work; medications were ineffective; destructive patterns continued. The professionals often gave up when it came to treating these clients, sending them away, saying, "Stop drinking, then I will work with you." In response to the collective abandonment by clinicians, Alcoholics Anonymous formed spontaneously when one *drunk* began helping another.

After an unsuccessful psychotherapy, Dr. Bob was lost to his continuing alcohol addiction. Through a chance meeting with Bill W., a conversation about addiction developed and a partnership dedicated to sobriety was formed. Dr. Bob and Bill W. talked at length about the effects of their addiction and used each other for mutual support in staying sober. Gradually, others joined them in talking about what they had been through and supporting each other's ongoing abstinence from alcohol. They formed a fellowship and wrote down the principles that allowed them to stay sober. The twelve steps became the foundation for sobriety for a wide range of addictions.

The twelve steps are the core of the Alcoholics Anonymous recovery program. (See Table 10-1.) The first step involves recognizing that you are powerless in relation to the addiction. This involves coming to terms with the fact that you cannot control the addiction, it is more powerful and cunning than you. In addition, the first step includes recognizing that the problem is out of hand and that life has become unmanageable because of the addiction. The second step recognizes that a higher power can help correct the insanity of addiction. Clients with an addiction try many things on their own to control or stop the addiction. This step suggests that it is impossible to do it yourself. You need the help of a higher power to recover. The third step involves an active decision to put your life in the hands of that higher power. Clients who are early in recovery from addiction may find it helpful to focus

Table 10-1 **The Twelve Steps of Alcoholics Anonymous**

1. We admitted we were powerless over alcohol—that our lives had be come unmanageable.

2. Came to believe that a Power greater than ourselves could restore us to sanity.

3. Made a decision to turn our will and our lives over to the care of God *as we understood Him.*

4. Made a searching and fearless moral inventory of ourselves.

5. Admitted to God, to ourselves and to another human being the exact nature of our wrongs.

6. Were entirely ready to have God remove all these defects of character.

7. Humbly asked Him to remove our shortcoming.

8. Made a list of all persons we had harmed, and became willing to make amends to them all.

9. Made direct amends to such people whenever possible, except when to do so would injure them or others.

10. Continued to take personal inventory and when we were wrong promptly admitted it.

11. Sought through prayer and meditation to improve our conscious contact with God, *as we understood Him,* praying only for knowledge of His will for us and the power to carry that out.

12. Having had a spiritual awakening as the result of these steps, we tried to carry this message to alcoholics, and to practice these principles in all our affairs.

The Twelve Steps are reprinted with permission of Alcoholics Anonymous World Services, Inc. Permission to reprint the Twelve Steps does not mean that A.A. has reviewed or approved the contents of this publication, nor that A.A. agrees with the views expressed herein. A.A. is a program of recovery from alcoholism only—use of the Twelve Steps in connection with programs and activities which are patterned after A.A., but which address other problems, or in any other non-A.A. context, does not imply otherwise.

on these three steps in treatment. The first three steps lay the necessary foundation for working in a recovery program—admitting there is a problem and asking for help from a higher power. For clients who are not particularly spiritual, the higher power may simply be the members of the anonymous recovery group.

The fourth step involves taking inventory of yourself. This means that you begin an ongoing process of honestly taking stock of your strengths and limitations. As you work with this fourth step, you give up both self-aggrandizing and self-deprecating perceptions. After taking an honest look at your strengths and limitations, the next step involves identifying when you were wrong and admitting it to others. The therapeutic process in this step is not only admitting what you have done wrong but in discussing it with others. This step recognizes the powerful therapeutic effect of talking about aspects of yourself that you may find shameful. The next steps involve asking for these shortcomings to be removed and making amends to anyone who has been harmed by those identified faults or actions. The last steps involve strengthening your awareness of a higher power to support recovery and encouraging the addict to take the message of recovery to others. The twelfth step lays the foundation for addicts in recovery to tell their stories to others, using the process of Dr. Bob and Bill W. to reinforce their own recovery and bring this method to others who need hope. In his story, Dr. Bob speculates about how sharing a discussion about recovery was helpful. He states, "He [Bill W.] gave me information about the subject of alcoholism, which was undoubtedly helpful. Of far more importance was the fact that he was the first living human with whom I had ever talked, who knew what he was talking about in regard to alcoholism from actual experience. In other words, he talked my language." (Anonymous, 1976.)

When someone attends a twelve-step group for the first time, they begin to work on the first step, which is admitting there is a problem with addiction. Meetings take place in space that is donated, usually in churches, schools, and sometimes hospitals. When you arrive at a meeting, you will generally find volunteers setting up chairs, literature, and coffee. Meetings begin with a reading of the preamble and the twelve steps. There is a recognition of newcomers and participants who have achieved significant milestones in their recovery, such as thirty days, sixty days, or one year of sobriety. At a *speakers meeting,* the body of the meeting is devoted to someone telling their story. They share their experiences of addiction and re-covery with the group. A *step meeting* will involve a discussion of one of the twelve steps. In addition, time is usually devoted to members sharing thoughts and experiences. The floor is left open for you to say whatever is on your mind. Members listen but do not give feedback. The response to someone speaking about what is on their mind is generally, "Thank you for shar-ing." Members are careful not to offer therapy to each other in meetings. The focus is on their personal work, not in fixing others. Each member is allowed to be where they are in their own recovery.

At its heart, this method involves both cognitive restruc-turing and spiritual awakening. The cognitive components of the program involve correcting distortions in thinking that ac-company addiction. Slogans and principles of recovery offer a type of reframing. The addict tends to develop a system of thinking that is built on denial and magical thinking. The twelve steps replace this addictive thinking with simple ideas that support sobriety, such as "Don't drink. Go to meetings." Many addicts develop a highly egocentric view of the world. They come to believe that they are the center of the universe and that the world revolves around them. Recognizing that there is something greater than yourself is a realistic cognitive shift. None of us is all powerful. By definition, being human involves some measure of powerlessness. Conversely, the opposite type of thinking distortion can occur. The addict may have so much shame and self-loathing that they believe they are the worst human being ever to live. Twelve-step programs can help you to see that others have had similar, if not worse, experiences during the active phases of their addictions. You are not the best or the worst, only human.

Some have speculated that the spiritual awakening is an integral part of recovery in the twelve-step programs. Bill W., AA's founder, believed that he could not have been successful in recovery without this process of enlightenment. For many people, increasing contact and awareness of a higher power has a powerful therapeutic effect. You can feel less alone. You can feel reassured that there is something to rely on when you are unable to fix everything yourself. You can give up trying to control all aspects of life and start to trust that there is some greater wisdom at work.

Twelve-step meetings are useful for decreasing shame. When an addict is feeling mortified about his symptoms and difficulties, guilt often keeps him from discussing addictive difficulties. At a twelve-step meeting, participants are open about having an addiction. There is no need for shame, because everyone at meetings struggles with common issues. The only requirement for membership is a desire to stop "using." Meetings offer a chance to see how others, via their success stories, have recovered from addiction. Modeling from peers can help the addict choose more adaptive patterns of coping. Members are encouraged to collaborate with someone in the group who has some experience with sobriety, or to find a sponsor. Sponsors help the person stay sober by offering support and sharing what has worked for them.

Twelve-step fellowship can be effective for a variety of addictive behaviors. However, there is a note of caution about the limitations of these methods with all addictive behaviors: This method can be helpful in counteracting urges to use alcohol and narcotics, however, effectiveness with cocaine addiction is more questionable. The urge to use cocaine tends to be episodic rather than continuous. Because cocaine is by nature a drug that involves bingeing, episodes of sobriety are often built into patterns of use. Urges to use cocaine can happen years after active use has ceased. The twelve-step method has also been used to control eating and sexual addictions. This is a more cumbersome application because abstinence from food and sex is not possible. Sexual perversion has roots deep in the personality. Recovery is not so easily achieved. Some counselors in Sex and Love Addicts Anonymous (SLAA) groups can have a precarious personality structure. They may not be the best models of well-adjusted sexuality.

In the past, twelve-step groups felt antagonistic about interventions from professional counselors. In addition, professional therapists were resistant to blending treatment in the office with support group meetings. This thankfully has changed. Now AA groups recognize that at times professional treatment is necessary and medications can play a role in recovery. Therapists recognize that the fellowship can offer support in a way that the therapist can't. Sponsors offer peer experience and twenty-four hour availability for support and interaction.

Perhaps the most remarkable feature of a twelve-step fellowship is that it is the only treatment that is absolutely free. No charge is ever levied to participants. You are welcome to come and take all the benefits of the program without ever contributing financially. No other treatment method can boast this type of benevolence or accessibility. Meetings are supported by volunteer donations, and a plate is usually passed around for collection.

Side Effects of Twelve-Step Groups

There may be some side effects to participation in a twelve-step program. A group can only progress as quickly as its slowest member. When people in recovery form groups, they bring a wide variety of personal styles and conflicts to the gathering. In general, groups tend to be positive. But members who are severely damaged may negatively influence the group's recovery. For example, if a group member develops active difficulty, the focus on this member might interfere with individual progress.

Twelve-step programs can become addictive in and of themselves. Some members will develop an overdependence on the twelve-step process. They may focus exclusively on the program and replace all their thinking with ideas from the twelve-step process. Although some dependence on the group and the process is necessary in the beginning, striking a balance is also important. Once sobriety is achieved, the structure of the fellowship program may become less needed in order to continue with a healthy life-style.

People in twelve-step groups believe that "once an addict, always an addict." Recovery is perpetual and never complete. The reason for embracing this value is because for many addicts, the risks associated with saying they are recovered are significant. If you think of yourself as cured, you might be tempted to try a controlled substance. Some people may be able to return to casual substance use, but for many addicts, continued use will be life-threatening. Although clinicians are not in agreement, perpetual recovery might be limiting in terms of personal development. Some clinicians believe that it is possible for some clients to achieve character change sufficient to eliminate the need for addiction symptoms. In other words, it may be possible to change to the extent that underlying conflicts which supported addictive behaviors no longer exist. The client can resolve the need to alter perceptions and emotions with substances. She can develop the ability to cope without using substances or addictive behaviors. However, other clinicians believe that to risk labeling this development as a cure is to risk relapse.

It is difficult to know who may be capable of this type of change. For other clients, the decision to abstain from substance use will be a conscious decision for the rest of their lives. The risk of lulling these clients into a false sense of security with an attitude that promotes controlled drinking or the idea that addiction can be cured is great. For this reason, twelve-step groups choose to say that recovery is ongoing, and the goal of abstinence is a prerequisite for membership. The idea that you can never be recovered might perpetuate a negative self-attitude and a feeling of being disordered or defective.

On the surface, the requirement for membership in a twelve-step group is simply the desire for sobriety. However, these groups have strong values and behavioral norms. Members are encouraged to adopt unquestioningly and implement the program's philosophy and beliefs. New members are encouraged to believe the tenets of the program on faith rather than critically evaluate these beliefs. The program suggests that addicts are poor judges about what is helpful and not helpful toward recovery. Indeed, the addict frequently exhibits impaired thinking when evaluating life-style choices. Independent thinking is what led the addict to his current difficulties. However, precisely because the addict is vulnerable to undue influence, his freedom to choose needs to be protected. Clients should be encouraged to evaluate a twelve-step program for a time-limited period to discern its effectiveness. Once sobriety is achieved, the validity of program tenets needs to be assessed for appropriateness in the client's recovery.

Bibliotherapy

Bibliotherapy involves reading books as a stimulus for personal development and growth. In any bookstore, one of the largest sections usually involves books devoted to self-help, covering almost every conceivable type of difficulty. Topics include relationships, specific diagnostic categories, relaxation, stress management, child rearing, anger, and intimacy. Recovery publications comprise a huge industry. You may find it helpful to simply browse the shelves and choose books that catch your interest. Whatever you need to learn will jump out from the other titles. Bibliotherapy is helpful in areas that are not highly conflicted. For example, if you have difficulty with time management, you may be able to solve it by reading a book about organizational skills. You might be able to implement keeping a date book and wearing a watch, with minimal effort. However, someone with addictive alcohol-use patterns will not be able to read a book about staying sober and just implement the changes. Getting sober is an experience and a behavior, not just acquiring information.

Bibliotherapy is particularly helpful if used in conjunction with consultation with a skilled care provider. A discussion of written material can provide useful grist for the mill in therapy sessions. Clients often bring in sections of books to share and express reactions to in-session. This is a valuable tool for developing new perspectives. Just last week, I noticed a client in the waiting room of our office, with a *DSM-IV* on his lap. I have no doubt that a lively discussion of diagnosis was a part of his session that day. Books can offer an excellent source of information, resources, and exercises.

Books cannot offer a substitute for a therapy relationship. Therapy takes place within the context of a relationship and involves interpersonal feedback. Reading is a passive, reflective process. Psychotherapy is a lived experience. However, information discovered in books may enhance the work of psychotherapy. What we learn in psychotherapy will make what we read more meaningful. There is a synergistic effect when bibliotherapy and psychotherapy are used together.

Journaling

Keeping a journal may be a useful support to the therapy process. Some people find the medium of writing—either electronically or on paper—to be comfortable and easy. It may be easier to express fears and fantasies in the privacy of your own writing. A journal may provide a more accurate record of symptoms as they occur in time. Writing down goals for your personal work can help keep you focused and may increase the likelihood of achieving goals. A journal can provide an ongoing account of your process. Often patterns may be easier to spot when recorded on paper. The journal may offer new perspectives when it is read again later. It is a way of giving yourself feedback about conflicts and issues. It can mark progress in treatment and illustrate accomplishments.

You may wish to deliberate about journaling and write at regularly scheduled intervals. Or you may wish to write whenever the inspiration strikes. You may wish to follow a structured form or simply write an account of your stream of consciousness. There are a number of commercially available guides to journaling. Some workbooks focus on specific exercises, which might include addiction issues, stress reduction, or working with dreams. For some people, following an unstructured writing process might feel more comfortable. All you need is paper and pen. Using special paper might stimulate creativity.

It is important that you feel secure that your journal is absolutely private. You are in control of who will share this information. If you do not live alone, find a place in which to lock your journal. Protect these self-disclosures so that you can feel safe to record your most unusual thoughts and intimate feelings. You may wish to bring parts of your journal into therapy sessions to discuss specific issues. Journaling requires that you find some quiet, private time to concentrate on writing. Carving out this type of personal time may in itself be therapeutic for people who are always busy.

If you wish to record a stream of consciousness, write in an unstructured fashion. Get comfortable; bring enough writing supplies so that you do not have to be interrupted. (For me this includes a beverage, as well as paper and pen.) When you are ready, try to write each thought that enters your mind. Do not criticize, judge, or edit. When you notice a critical thought such as "This is stupid" or "I can't write," observe it, and note it with interest. Where did these critical ideas come from? Teachers? Parents? Write to express your feelings. Write to record your ideas. Write to remember insights and patterns you're aware of. You may wish to write about feelings and developments in the therapy process. A journal can provide a place to extend the work that occurs in-session. This is particularly true if the journal is brought into sessions and sections are understood together with the therapist.

Hypnosis

Clinical use of hypnosis has a long and respected tradition. Hypnosis is a relaxed state where the mind can be open to ideas and suggestions. Hypnosis involves relaxing the mind by focusing on specific stimuli. It may be accomplished through progressive muscle relaxation or visualization of a relaxing image. It may involve focusing attention inward on breathing or on an outer object, such as a flame. The mind is quieted and can be open to exploration and recollection of memories or may be more receptive to suggestion.

Hypnosis may be useful in helping you deal with anxiety or fears. Essentially, hypnosis is a profound state of relaxation. Physiologically, it is impossible for the body to be relaxed and anxious simultaneously. When a person reaches a relaxed state through hypnosis, ideas that stimulate anxiety may be examined and altered. For example, suggestions about feeling confident or coping with fear may be made during hypnosis. The mind is more open to these suggestions because anxiety does not interfere with incorporating this information. In a state of hypnosis, a person may be able to imagine some previously feared situation, such as public speaking, and visualize coping adequately with the anxiety. Even if suggestions or visualizations are not used, the act of achieving a profoundly relaxed state may be beneficial. Practice reinforces the ability to quickly reach a relaxed state, and this can be used in everyday situations.

Hypnosis is also used by some therapists to facilitate exploration of past-life experiences. This process has been surprisingly helpful for some clients. Perhaps the most fascinating account of the discovery of past-life regression therapy is in Brian Weiss's classic work *Many Lives, Many Masters*. In the course of his work as a psychotherapist, Weiss discovered that clients using hypnosis were able to recall events from other lifetimes. Once these lives were recalled, present-day symptoms were resolved and disappeared.

This phenomenon does not fall into the mainstream practice of psychology or psychiatry. Most therapists would agree that beliefs about past incarnations fall into the realm of spirituality rather than ordinary psychological functioning. However, the astute therapist might be alert to evidence that these beliefs affect the client, and work with him in whatever way is useful.

Emerging Therapies

New treatments are always being researched and investigated. Often, the most talented clinicians in the field are developing new ways to assist in alleviating symptoms. These bright forward thinkers offer exciting perspectives that advance our understanding. New ideas need to be carefully evaluated before they are widely implemented. Clinicians attempt to validate theories with empirical research. New treatments can be studied to evaluate efficacy, side effects, and indications for use.

Adjunct Therapies

There are wonderful opportunities for self-healing, self-exploration, and self-soothing through adjunct therapies including art, music, movement, dance therapy, and psychodrama. The arts offer a form for expression of the self. If you observe the self as it is expressed, you will learn about psychological and emotional functioning. All artistic expression involves a projection of mental life. Through the arts, we can learn to interpret psychological processes as they are observed in movement, sound, color, or shape.

Art

Art therapy involves using art to resolve emotional difficulties, as well as better know your inner mental world. Artistic expression can be cathartic. Emotions that cannot be released verbally may find expression in color or shape through paint or clay. Art may be calming to frazzled nerves. It can be a focus of concentration that allows a person to forget anxious worries. Art does not have to mean classical painting or sculpting. It might be crocheting or dance. Creating art is therapeutic.

Music Therapy

It seems intuitive to talk about the soothing and therapeutic effects of music. Science is slowly catching up with intuition, and the therapeutic benefits of music are being documented with empirical data. Listening to music can evoke emotional responses. Playing music can help you connect with your higher power.

Movement Therapy

We are dynamic, moving beings. We are rarely still. Conscious use of movement can alter how we feel. We can understand more about how we feel by increasing awareness of our nonverbal behaviors and messages. Participation in dance can be an emotional expression. Movement benefits the cardiovascular and musculoskeletal systems. Clients can achieve movement goals to increase a sense of mastery and accomplishment.

Dance Therapy

Dance therapy involves the specific use of dance to resolve emotional difficulties. It is particularly useful if conflicts have their origins in nonverbal developmental phases. For example, expression of primitive emotions in the medium of dance may allow visceral resolution of conflicts and experiential healing. In addition to expressive benefits of dance, there may be direct physiological benefits. Movement and activity can improve mood. Music, when combined with movement, can be prescribed to produce optimal results.

Psychodrama

Psychodrama is a unique form of therapy that involves working through difficulties via extemporaneous performance but with structured rules and techniques. Roles can be assigned to members of the group, and aspects of a situation or conflict can be worked through with a group think. The therapist is active and serves as a director; she stops scenes and inquires about feelings, assigns roles, and suggests dialogue. Clients enjoy this form of treatment, which requires a great effort of energy and a degree of comfort with group sharing.

Pet Therapy

A surprisingly valuable mode of adjunct therapy is working with animals. It is particularly useful for geriatric clients, as interacting with animals combines physical movement and emotional stimulation. During the course of my work at a local state institution for the chronically mentally ill, we used to take clients to a farm to make use of activities such as hayrides and picking pumpkins. The farm had a section for petting animals. One overcast fall day, we took the clients for an afternoon outing. Heywood, a client with a thirty-five-year history of chronic paranoid schizophrenia, accompanied me to the petting area. This area contained donkeys, pigs, sheep, rabbits, chickens, a goat, and several docile cows. Heywood, a man of few words, was bothered almost all the time by hallucinations of hands in front of his face, taunting him. In the hospital, he frequently boxed in the air with these hallucinatory hands. He mumbled most times in a characteristically incoherent fashion. Although Heywood was six foot three inches tall and weighed two hundred and eighty pounds, at heart he was a gentle person. He responded warmly to smiles, with grin of his own. Heywood came upon the cows, chewing away in their pen. He walked up to one cow, and said, "Hello. How are you today?" He then leaned his forehead onto the forehead of the cow, and stood conversing casually but meaningfully with this animal. When he finished, he thanked the cow, wished her a good day, and ambled on to find the rest of the group. Heywood, who rarely conversed with people, had been able to have a satisfying conversation with this large, docile animal.

Alternative Therapies

There is a growing interest in alternative health care methods by clinicians, researchers, and the National Institutes of Health. This increased interest allows us to explore how complementary practices can improve our mental health.

Acupuncture has long been used to treat anxiety and depression. However, we must keep in mind that the traditional Chinese medical view of anxiety and depression is radically different from our Western understanding. They view emotional states as arising from physical states or imbalances in chi. Even given these philosophical differences, acupuncture can offer a safe, effective method for treating difficult emotional states.

Herbalists are well aware of the powerful psychoactive

effects of the plants. Herbs can profoundly affect mood, energy, and feelings. But they must be used with knowledge and caution. A naturopathic physician or nutritionist can help guide your choices in the use of herbs or vitamin supplements. As with medications, herbs should be used only when necessary and in the lowest doses possible. There are a number of herbal supplements being investigated for their specific effects. One example is ginkgo, which is being studied for its effects on circulation to the brain. The increased circulation seems to have a positive effect on alertness, mental efficiency, and memory, and some clinicians are hopeful that ginkgo may be useful in the treatment of dementia. Other herbs under investigation include ginseng, St. John's Wort, chamomile, catnip, and valerian. Special diets, such as macrobiotics, are also being studied for their effects on energy and mood.

In addition to these alternatives, other forms of treatment including aromatherapy, meditation, and massage have been shown to improve mood, coping abilities, and relaxation. Used appropriately, complementary methods and alternative practices can improve our mental and emotional well-being.

CHAPTER 11

Natural Therapy

N atural human experience offers therapeutic effects. Events that take place in life and relationships with others can provide opportunities for personal growth, behavioral change, and resolution of conflicts. Changes in routine and life-style may provide an optimal environment for stimulating growth. For example, you may have felt the positive, therapeutic effects of taking a vacation. Time off can provide opportunities for introspection. After spending several days in quiet reflection on the beach or in the forest, we can feel renewed energy and a more directed purpose. Life presents experiences that naturally help us grow, resolve conflicts, and heal inner turmoil. Therapy need not always be clinical. It occurs in the natural order of experience.

Some experiences that are naturally therapeutic include meditation, relationships, and learning. Life-style changes can have a profound impact on psychological well-being including nutrition, exercise, and relaxation. Spirituality is naturally healing, as is contact with nature. These life experiences can be beneficial either alone or in conjunction with psychotherapy.

Growth and Development

The natural patterns of growth and development provide a method for increasing adjustment and adaptation. Growth involves biological maturation and learning through experiences. As we grow physically, our bodies acquire new abilities to think and move. We become capable of complex, sustained, directed activities with gradually acquired abilities. In infancy we cannot even move ourselves within our environment. We develop to be able to accomplish a wide range of psychomotor behaviors, including playing sports or musical instruments, conducting surgery, discovering scientific theories, or flying a plane. Our experiences challenge us to use our abilities in new ways.

Robert Kegan, a developmental psychologist at Harvard University, blended the work of Piaget and Freud. He constructed a model of development that suggests natural development of skills and capacities through normal process of growth, maturation, and experience. As we grow physically, we become capable of experiencing greater challenges. With experience, we develop methods of coping with a wide array of challenges. As we grow we become capable of more, and we are inspired to learn by venturing out into the world. As we exercise our capacities, they expand. Our natural developmental process is directed toward achieving wisdom and optimal adaptation.

Life Experiences

Experiences that occur in life can produce many of the same results as psychotherapy. For example, therapy can affirm our identity. Getting a job after a tough interview or receiving a diploma can have the same effect. Therapy can offer support.

Friendships and love relationships can offer similar experiences.

Experiences help to shape our personality. We form a sense of ourselves through evaluating our abilities. When the world gives us praise for what we are able to accomplish, we will form an opinion of ourselves as capable. We will carry these experiences of mastery into new situations and be able to trust that although we may not have met this particular challenge before, we know we can successfully meet it. The importance of allowing the developing child to have mastery experiences cannot be underemphasized. The child must see others delighted in his early abilities. When you are able to celebrate accomplishments, including vocalizations and psychomotor tasks, such as building with blocks or crawling, the child begins to celebrate his own abilities. A sense of confidence begins.

Experiences can also shape our adult development. It is not necessarily true that "that which does not kill us makes us stronger." Sometimes we are injured in the process of trauma. For example, if something traumatic happens to us, such as the death of a loved one or an injury, we learn about life's potential negative experiences. If we are spared these experiences, we may be spared some of the harsh possibilities of human experience. Positive experiences, such as parenting, will expand your abilities through a range of new challenges. Having work or professional successes may reinforce one's sense of identity and capability.

Sometimes learning takes place through trial and error. At other times we learn by watching what happens to other people. When you have experiences, such as raising children, you learn about yourself by incurring new experiences or relationships and by gaining perspective from another vantage point. We can share our learnings with others through the process of teaching.

Meditation

Meditation is the process of focusing the mind on quiet thoughts and allowing for peace of mind. It may involve focusing on a sound, color, even a flame. You can experience a simple meditation by taking a moment to focus on your breath. You may wish to focus on the rising and falling of your abdomen as you inhale and exhale. Or you may focus on the feeling of the air at your nostrils as you inhale and exhale. Focus on your breathing, and gently release any other thoughts. If you notice another thought, gently bring back your focus to your breathing. Gradually, the space between thoughts will increase and you will be able to be aware of the space that is in between everything. This space of existence is the higher power. It is the context for all thoughts and actions, and when we are quiet, we can be aware of this awesome energy.

It may be helpful to set aside ten or fifteen minutes twice a day for meditation practice. Results may be evident immediately or may occur gradually. It is best to approach meditation without any preconceived expectations. Try it and see what develops. See if you find the experience beneficial in the long run, without judging each individual session. Do not strive to become a "good meditator." Just see what happens.

Meditation can allow you to be in the space between the thoughts. It increases your awareness of the space that supports existence. We end up focusing most of our mental activity on our thoughts. Meditation offers a refreshing break from this vigilance. Through quieting the mind of its usual clamor, you can begin to have a pure experience of existence. Sometimes there is an awareness of being connected to a universal energy or space through meditation. A sense of peace, well-being, and calm may develop with the practice over time.

Meditation is particularly beneficial for clients who are anxious or troubled by stress. Surprisingly, clients with addictive difficulties often may benefit from the practice of regular meditation.

Relationships

Humans are social beings by nature. Satisfying relationships can sustain us through the most trying circumstances. There is comfort in the nearness of others, in sharing fears and anxieties. We learn about ourselves through our relationships.

In intimacy, we see ourselves reflected back. We experience the satisfaction of having another person who says, "I accept you as you are." We feel comfortable sharing all of ourselves with another, secure that we will not be shamed.

Our relationships give us feedback about who we are. We see ourselves mirrored in the reflections of our interactions with others. To some extent, we create our interactions in order to satisfy relationship needs.

Learning

Human beings seem to have an innate thirst for knowledge. From the moment we begin to explore ourselves and our world, we are intent on learning. Through study we are exposed to a variety of ways of thinking. We share complex human experiences and learn from the experiences of others. If relationships trouble us, we can learn techniques of communication. If we are curious about symptoms, we may study mental functioning. We can learn about physical and biological functioning, as well as emotions and temperament.

Learning new ideas can produce a sense of relief as new perspectives are encountered. If we learn about others in a similar situation, our sense of isolation is decreased. We may feel less alone when we read an author who shares their personal experiences.

Life-style

Our fundamental approach to life has an impact on our psychological well-being. If we clearly embrace the responsibility to influence life's satisfaction, adjustment may be more adaptive. If we are able to make decisions that enhance feelings of well-being, we may develop a sense of control and mastery about our lives. We develop an internal locus of control and take responsibility for influencing our own destiny. Unfortunately in this society, it is a myth that we will be cared for by others if we become unable to care for ourselves. Wishes for dependency gratification are likely to be disappointed. Doctors can't care for you; nurses can't make it all better. At best, restoration of well-being will be a partnership, with equal (but different) contributions from both participants. A healthy life-style involves attention to biological, psychological, social, and spiritual well-being.

The old saying, "everything in moderation" may be familiar, but it is a useful guide for a balanced life-style. Life's ordinary distresses may be better managed, if excessive behaviors do not produce additional stress.

Nutrition

Food affects mood, according to new studies. Foods like pasta can improve energy available to cope with emotional difficulties, as well as medical difficulties. The role of nutrition has long been recognized in medical treatment. It makes sense that emotional recovery can be supported by proper diet. Evidence about vitamins is mixed. Old ideas about vitamin therapy have fallen out of favor, but balanced nutritional habits can add to homeostasis. Vitamins are best received from foods. Increasing evidence about the benefits of herbs are being recognized by Western medical researchers. Herbs should be used with respect, as they can have all the side effects of medications if used improperly. Herbs are powerful compounds.

The human body needs a variety of nutrients to perform at its best. Most of us are aware that food choices can affect our energy level. Perhaps we have felt the urge to take a nap after the traditional Thanksgiving turkey meal, or have experienced a release from sluggishness after eating fruits and vegetables. However, many people are surprised to discover that food can also affect our mood. New research suggests that food choices can influence feelings of depression and anxiety. Medical studies on the impact of vitamins have led to an understanding of the effects of malnutrition, as well as identified positive benefits to a balanced consumption of these nutrients.

One method for improving eating habits is to become increasingly aware of food choices. Much of our food choosing goes on below the level of consciousness as we respond to habits and impulses. Awareness can create an opportunity for honoring the body by providing adequate nurturing. Eating well can be a physical, cellular affirmation of body functioning. Learn what balance in amounts and types of food is optimally and uniquely yours. Start by assessing current naturally occurring patterns by simply recording what you eat. At the end of several days, review where changes can be made. Develop a pattern of eating that is tailored to your life-style. Be creative, and enjoy food choices. Use herbs and spices to excite your appetite!

Generally accepted recommendations for diet include increasing consumption of fruits and vegetables, as well as whole grains. Four to six servings of fruits and vegetables are considered optimal. Fresh and whole foods are best. Wash vegetables thoroughly so that you remove traces of dirt, fertilizer, and pesticides. Four servings of whole grains can be included in breads, pasta, and rice dishes. Protein, such as fish and meats, should be eaten in moderation. Decreasing intake of fats and sugars is believed to reduce risks of many diseases.

The human body is 70 percent fluid. Each cell is composed of fluids, which plays an important role in feelings of well-being; daily intake should be at least two liters, unless contraindicated by a physician's orders due to clinical conditions. Fluid is essential to assist the body in removing toxic wastes through the kidneys and the skin. So what is two liters? How does this recommendation translate into action? How can you drink eight glasses of water, tea, juice, or milk? Ask for a glass of water with each meal. Alcohol should not be considered a fluid because it has a diuretic effect, and is not readily absorbed into the system.

Balanced Activity

We have learned that balanced activity is important in promoting overall health. Regular exercise improves cardiovascular functioning and strengthens muscles. It decreases bone loss due to aging. Exercise releases natural opiatelike substances (endorphins and enkephalins), which increase a sense of comfort. Psychologically, achieving physical goals can increase a sense of ability in addressing life's problems. Over the past century, our work has shifted from physical to intellectual. As our activity at work has decreased, we have shifted our focus during leisure hours to include the exercise of our physical abilities. To achieve our highest potential, our lifestyle must include some provisions for athletic activity. As the saying goes, "Use it or lose it."

Children have a natural love of exercising their physical capabilities. They run and jump spontaneously with natural delight. We have to *teach* children to "sit still" and use their energy for concentration rather than activity. Starting in elementary school, physical activities have become a part of the mandatory curriculum. Many children start to participate in organized physical activities as a natural extension of play. Feelings about physical ability and the capacity to enjoy physical activity are deeply embedded in development and self-concept. Mastery of physical and sports skills can boost self-esteem. When activity is encouraged and enjoyed in childhood, it may be easier to incorporate an exercise program into adult, working life-styles. The simplest form of exercise is walking. Or you may wish to find forms of activity that are more recreational, such as tennis, golf, or volleyball.

The benefits of exercise become readily apparent almost immediately upon beginning a fitness program. Regular exercise improves muscular strength, endurance, flexibility, and cardiovascular efficiency. Exercise lowers the resting heart rate and allows the heart to more easily carry nutrients to cells and remove waste from body cells. Exercise reduces blood-cholesterol levels, bone loss due to aging, feelings of anxiety and depression, chronic fatigue, and insomnia. A regular activity schedule lowers body weight by burning calories and suppressing appetite and increasing the rate of absorption and use of food. In addition, exercise improves appearance and self-image.

Although many people have already adopted a program of regular exercise, some people have difficulty establishing a pattern of regular activity. Feelings of fatigue or unworthiness may inhibit our motivation. The demands of everyday living may appear to have priority over exercise.

Sleep

The body restores and repairs itself during sleep. Growth and regeneration require sleep. Sleep is necessary for emotional stability and equanimity. There is no universal *proper* amount of sleep. Individual patterns vary with age, physiological needs, and scheduling demands. Find the pattern that helps you to have the most available energy. To promote the formation of patterns sleep and get up at regular times. This appears to strengthen the body's natural twenty-four-hour rhythm and leads to the regular onset of sleep at night. Exercise in steady, daily amounts may help to deepen sleep over the long term. It is best to exercise early in the day to avoid getting energized immediately before trying to get to sleep. Create an optimal environment for sleep. Block out loud noises by wearing earplugs or by creating neutral background noise. Sleep in a cool (not cold) room. Excessive warmth may also disrupt sleep.

Don't try to sleep when you are hungry. Eating a light bedtime snack may induce drowsiness. Foods high in tryptophan seem to promote sleep. These include warm or cold milk, whole wheat, eggs, and turkey. Avoid the use of tryptophan supplements, as they have been linked to long-term complications. Avoid caffeine in the afternoon and evening, as it stays in your system for up to twelve hours. If you drink alcohol, do so only in moderation and early in the evening. Nightcaps may help you fall asleep but they lead to more fragmented sleep with more awakenings.

It is best to avoid the chronic use of sleeping pills. Occasional use may be beneficial, but chronic use of hypnotics may be ineffective and detrimental for some people with insomnia. Discuss the use of melatonin preparations with your physician. The use of these hormone supplements is new, and further testing is necessary before conclusions about safety can be considered reliable.

If you can't fall asleep after trying for a half hour, don't stay in bed. Get up and try again when you are tired. If worries and thoughts keep you from falling asleep, keep a pen and paper at your bedside. Write down any concerns, then let them go. Allow the list to keep track of worries for you until morning.

Relaxation

Stress is inherent in the human experience. Indeed, we are biologically wired to adapt to stress as a mechanism to ensure survival. Stress-related disorders appear to be epidemic in our modern society. Some stress is helpful in that it motivates us to make changes and improve our lives. Reactions to stress may heighten our sense of need and prompt us to find ways to satisfy any unmet needs. However, the destructive effects of prolonged stress, even in moderate amounts, can limit our optimal experience of well-being.

Developing a program of stress management promises many physiological, psychological, emotional, and spiritual benefits. In addition to fitness training, a program of stress management can include meditation, socializing with friends or family, participating in entertainment, or enjoying nature. As discussed, exercise, nutrition, and sleep play an important role in coping with stress. Exercise is a natural method of releasing tension in muscles. Getting adequate sleep and rest will help reenergize the body. Eating a balanced diet will provide fuel and energy for body and mind. It is best to eliminate or restrict the amount of alcohol, caffeine, and other mood-altering substances used as a means of managing stress.

Improving time-management skills may reduce a sense of pressure or urgency in your day. Perhaps it would be helpful to get out of bed a few minutes earlier in order to have more time to prepare for the day. Using time to its optimal potential may increase your sense of control and organization. Structure and habits reduce stress.

Our perceptions significantly influence our experience of stress. If we can learn to view *failures* as opportunities for growth, we conserve energy for constructive use. Rather than harshly condemning yourself and others, find ways to work constructively on perceived shortcomings. We are, at best, a work in progress. Develop an optimistic view of the world, and try to see the best in people. You may wish to do something for others so that you can take your mind off yourself and boost your self-esteem.

Developing techniques for assertiveness may increase a sense of personal control. It may be helpful to learn to recognize your personal rights, as well as set boundaries on the demands of others. A support system of colleagues and like-minded friends can bolster personal resources and validate personal experiences. We can all benefit from talking with someone who shares our experiences and who can say, "I see it exactly the way you do."

Finding opportunities to laugh releases tension and relaxes mind and body. The health benefits of laughter are currently being explored. Laughter appears to promote optimal brain chemistry and may support the release of healing neurotransmitters and hormones. Developing a sense of humor that allows you to let go of the seriousness of a situation can help you through even the most difficult circumstances.

You may wish to learn relaxation techniques (breathing, progressive relaxation, or visualization) to release tension and quiet your mind. The benefits of meditation have been taught for thousands of years. Any method for quieting the mind will prove helpful in coping with stress. Forms of meditation include sitting meditation, focusing on a sound or phrase, walking meditation, or awareness meditation. Singing and praying are natural forms of meditation. There is an exciting variety of commercially prepared audio- and videotapes to guide meditation sessions. Experiment with what makes you feel the best.

When you are experiencing an unusual amount of stress, it may be helpful to develop a plan of care that can restore equilibrium. Treat yourself as if you have a *situational* flu, and implement self-help treatments, such as extra fluids and rest, and chicken or vegetable soup. Take extra precautions while driving a motor vehicle, as you may be easily distracted. Be aware of alcohol intake and the amount of smoking, as both habits may be easy to overdo as a result of stress. If eating is a coping mechanism, keep a journal of food intake so that when you are experiencing stress, any extra food consumption will be easily recognized. If specialized types of stress reduction and coping strategies are to be used, it may be most helpful to learn them from expert clinicians.

Spirituality

Awareness of our spirituality can have a powerful life-enhancing effect. Having a connection to a higher power can increase a person's sense of security and energy for life. Often, a connection to a higher power or God presence fosters a sense of being connected to a whole, of being at one with all that is in existence. Faith in God can help us to believe that there is some reasoning behind events that occur, and that good will prevail over evil.

Some clinicians liken karma to the psychoanalytic process of understanding the unconscious. Seeing patterns of actions and consequences can help us understand the meaning and purpose in our lives. Some believe that Zen practice is an extension of psychoanalytic method, or vice versa. In Zen meditation, thoughts form a type of free association, and are let go as the mind is quieted.

Believing in a higher power may offer a sense of being nurtured or guided. We often view God with a parental interpretation. We may understand events and communications in prayer as offering guidance about choices. The sense that we are not alone in our decisions can be comforting. Spiritual beliefs guide our conduct in physical life. If we are able to invoke a loving image of God, we may feel comforted in times of distress. In the words of Voltaire, if God didn't exist, man would have to invent him.

Contact with Nature

For many people, contact with nature is therapeutic. If we can find places where nature is in abundance, we can begin to feel renewed from the energy of the earth. We feel the wind and become part of the sky. Feeling the rhythms of nature can restore a sense of order in an otherwise chaotic world. In our increasingly technological world, we easily become removed from nature. The reality of cyberspace must be balanced with feeling the spray of an ocean or a mountain breeze.

It is also therapeutic to have contact with animals, which reminds us of the variety that is possible. It calls us to be curious about our relationship with these creatures and to wonder about our own origins. We are reminded of our own basic instincts by watching animal behavior.

Nature follows a pattern of recycling and conserving. Time has natural rhythms. Growth of one part has an impact on all the parts in a system. Birth and death follow a natural order and allow for strengthening the species. Having contact with the rhythms and cycles of nature can remind us of our own inherent cycles.

CHAPTER 12

What to Avoid in Therapy

People in distress are vulnerable. Distress is a powerful motivator. When a treatment promises relief, and other methods have failed, you may be motivated to try unorthodox approaches. Judgment about choices in therapy may be compromised because of a pressing need to obtain relief. A client may be more easily coerced into participating in treatments that appear to offer faster, more effective relief. The professional therapist has an obligation to protect the client from entering into relationships that may be exploitive.

Avoid Distance Therapy: Radio Call-in/Talk Shows, Virtual Therapy Sessions

Clients often ask me what I think about on-air psychotherapists. Some radio psychotherapists offer useful informational programs. Call-in programs, however, begin to carry some risks. Some hosts of these shows are licensed professionals; some are not. For example, one on-air psychotherapist is often critical and judgmental of callers. She often suggests that people stop focusing on the past and simply get on with life. This advice may seem attractive, but it may be impossible to follow. Symptoms sometimes keep people from being able to simply move forward. In listening closely to this radio therapist, she is careful to state that her ideas should not be applied to "clinical conditions." On closer examination, her credentials are seriously suspect. She makes it known that hers is an advice column, not a treatment format.

It is unethical, if not illegal, for a therapist to imply that they are doing treatment on the radio or on television, since an accurate assessment of mental health difficulties needs to be individualized and takes time. A therapist cannot make an accurate diagnosis or formulate an individualized treatment plan on the basis of a brief description of some difficulty, which is offered without the benefit of a private session. The purpose of a talk show is entertainment. Therapists on the radio have a legal responsibility to make clear that they are entertaining the public, not treating it.

Some clinicians are beginning to investigate techniques that involve computer technology. Interactive programs have been developed to mimic aspects of the psychotherapy relationship. Some of these programs have a clinical, scientific basis. For example, attempts to create an interactive diagnostic interview using the *DSM-IV* criteria have been made. This interactive program asks a series of questions about symptoms and manifestations of a disorder and then codes responses to offer a tentative diagnosis. The questions are based on a well-developed diagnostic tool that has been used manually for years and has been shown to be reliable and valid. This may have some usefulness to triage large numbers of patients and ensure a complete assessment, as well as supplement a face-to-face interview. Other programs are developed for entertainment or education purposes.

With the increasing popularity of the Internet, therapists may offer services across the Web. Even when a qualified therapist offers these services, virtual therapy lacks several essential elements of psychotherapy. For example, virtual therapy does not allow for face-to-face contact. Dynamic psychotherapy assumes an interpersonal relationship and provides a context for the psychological work. Even when a therapy has a behavioral focus, the real presence of the therapist often provides much-needed support. Virtual forms of therapy may offer contact with the therapist through a bulletin board or private chat room. This allows for a real-time dialogue, in writing, with some expression of nonverbals, learned as a part of the language of the Internet. However, significant information through nonverbal communication is lost. People use information from nonverbal interactions to clarify communications and obtain feedback.

The most significant danger in virtual therapy is that there is no way to verify the credentials of someone posing as a therapist. Some psychologists communicating on the Web attempt to remedy this by displaying curriculum vitae and licensing information. However, regulations about what types of information can be posted are slow in coming. Limits on what individuals can say are in conflict with the first amendment. There is a difficulty in regulating information available on the Internet because it is a global enterprise. There is a risk that unsuspecting users of a virtual therapy service will be taking advice from someone who is not qualified to address serious mental health concerns. In addition, there is no way to follow up with interactions over the Web. Evaluating the impact of interventions is an essential part of the therapy relationship.

Legitimate Internet sites that offer interaction with a qualified psychotherapist are being developed. These sites provide easily accessible information for consumers. In the future, protected sites might be created to allow for increased individual attention, full evaluation, and ongoing monitoring. Research is necessary to evaluate the impact of the potential benefits and drawbacks of virtual therapy.

Avoid Fads

It may be difficult to distinguish between what might be a promising new theory or treatment and what is a popular cultural fad. For example, in Vienna, late 1880s, it became trendy to seek psychoanalysis as a form of self-exploration. One way to evaluate an idea or treatment is to learn about the rationale and studies that support the approach. Compare this rationale with mainstream or conventional approaches. Do the ideas offer some additional perspective to current understandings? How consistent with previous evidence are the new ideas?

When an intervention or theory rests too heavily on the idea of one person, charismatic delivery, or an inspirational message, the theory is less likely to be able to withstand scientific scrutiny. When many clinicians have contributed to ideas and evaluated practice methods, data are more available to support ongoing use if a treatment is effective. Collaboration on the results of interventions allows a body of knowledge to develop about when and with whom treatment is likely to be effective, and also about potential side effects.

In evaluating ideas that I consider to be faddish or have little clinical merit, I am aware that for some individuals there are often positive results. Every therapy needs to be evaluated on the basis of whether it works. If it works, do it. Nonetheless, some trends in psychotherapy that have come and gone include inner child work, EST workshops, hydrotherapy, primal scream therapy, and even some biological treatments, such as megavitamin therapy.

Avoid Unrealistic Promises

If it seems too good to be true, it probably is. A treatment that promises to deliver unrealistic results has a greater likelihood of disappointing clients. The goals of treatment interventions need to be within the capabilities of the client, given the support and nature of the therapy. Change is usually accomplished gradually—with repeated practice—and over time. The longer that symptoms have been present and the more severe the symptom, the more difficult it may be to remove it. Be wary of therapies that promise to deliver significant behavioral change with little effort. For example, a dedicated couch potato cannot become a marathon runner overnight.

Sometimes in therapy, significant improvement and relief are experienced almost immediately. Quick results may happen. Insights may have a huge impact on behavior and lifestyle. When goals are set within the ability of the client, achievements can be seen at regular intervals. One example of unrealistic goals can be found in a self-help group designed to support members in pursuit of everlasting physical life. They report to have developed a method to help you prolong physical life forever. If you join, you can learn the secrets to everlasting youth. One drawback is that everlasting youth comes at a sizable fee. Common sense tells us that living forever is not possible. After all, no one ever *has* lived forever. It will be interesting to see the effects on this self-help group as the movement's leaders age and pass away themselves.

Avoid Poorly Skilled Clinicians

Avoid untrained clinicians. You must evaluate the therapist's qualifications to practice. Find out what education and licensing preparation the therapist has completed. Although legitimate credentials are not a guarantee of competency, licenses provide some measure of minimal competence for acceptable practice.

There is a wide variation in the abilities of therapists who successfully complete licensing and educational requirements for practice. In addition to formal credentials, you must personally evaluate the therapist's competence. Evaluate the therapist's clinical experience and ask about previous work with similar difficulties. Evaluate the match between you and your therapist. Periodically review goals to assess progress.

A therapist who is poorly trained to handle serious mental health difficulties may inadvertently inflict harm on clients. Therapists have an ethical and legal responsibility to maintain competence within the areas they practice and to practice only in areas and with methods for which they have been specifically trained.

If you find yourself in a situation with someone who does not seem able to help you, discuss your concerns with your therapist. You and your therapist may decide that an additional opinion may be helpful in clarifying treatment goals and approaches. An ethical therapist should feel confident in requesting a consultation from a colleague at anytime. The therapist should facilitate consultation upon a client's request, or when a need for additional information is recognized. If a therapist is defensive about discussing work with a colleague or becomes secretive about the treatment, this is a warning signal. You and your therapist should feel comfortable examining the process in the light of a well-lit room, with a consultant who is qualified.

The quality of therapy is difficult to evalute because on its face, therapy is just talking. The things that make ordinary talking and therapy different may be difficult to identify to the unskilled eye. Because it's just talking, many people believe they can do it. It is true that a layperson can mimic a therapist easily, asking, "How does that make you feel?" and mumbling "hmmm" at various times. To suggest that this is therapy is tantamount to believing that someone who can use a knife and fork can do surgery. It is a false belief that because you are capable of converstaion, you are capable of therapy. The talking cure is a complex process that requires a skilled mental surgeon.

For example, in one drug-treatment facility, *counselors* had little formal education about clinical treatment. One counselor was the janitor by day (buffing the kitchen floors) and the therapist by night (running groups for recovering addicts). This counselor had no formal education and limited supervision from the facility. Clients in this rehab were newly off of substances, incurring all the raw neurological experiences of being drug-free for less than forty-eight hours. This therapist would take newly drug-free clients into a group at night and sit one person in the center of a circle, and goad or badger them to "break down" and share their feelings. He would force clients to talk about painful experiences during the neurochemical upheaval that accompanies early sobriety. Not only are people incapable of processing emotions in a useful fashion at this stage, but they were retraumatized by reliving painful emotions.

There are no guarantees in therapy, as there are no guarantees in medical treatment. Succes depends on a number of factors, including effort put forth by the client and therapist. Don't believe promises of bliss, nirvana, or everlasting peace. Life just isn't built that way. The goal of therapy is to replace misery with common, ordinary unhappiness.

Avoid Quick Fixes

Avoid treatments that promise an instant cure. Treatment often takes time. It always takes effort. Promises of instant cures are likely to disappoint the client. For example, it is impossible to change basic personality in a weekend workshop. It is possible in a weekend workshop to access emotionally painful memories, but this type of sudden access may be overwhelming for some clients. Traumatic experiences need to be reworked in an environment that provides emotional safety, such as the context of ongoing psychotherapy. If you have a lifetime of abusive experiences to come to terms with, don't expect to do so in a weekend. It may have taken years to get to this point, so it will take time to heal. Healing is a process, not an event. Do not expect lightning bolts or earth-shattering experiences. Clients often have the misconception that they will find a single cause for their dysfunction. They expect to trace personality to a single event in development. Personality is a result of the totality of experience, a multidetermined dynamic process that cannot be traced to a single etiology.

The mind is complex. Psychological distress usually isn't simple. Respect the nature of the mind, and go gently toward recovery. Quick symptom removal carries the risk of disrupting emotional equilibrium. For example, depression may be covering a more serious symptom process. Depression can serve to quiet and simplify a mind that was before overwhelmed with anxiety and thought distortions. It may be better to understand the nature of the depression before removing and discarding it.

The need for emotional safety in order to explore symptoms and past experiences cannot be underestimated. The client's ego needs to know that it can process any emotions that may occur and that ordinary mental functioning will not be overwhelmed. The climate of trust that is necessary for deep exploration often takes more than a year to accomplish. Clients begin exploration in layers and periodically revisit issues that are significant, with new perspectives and insights. As the client explores, the therapist assists with labeling emotions, clarifying conflicts, and identifying dynamic patterns. In so doing, the client masters the memory of the painful experiences rather than being retraumatized with the retelling.

In some clients, quickly reexperiencing emotional traumas may be too painful to bear. At the end of the workshop, a client may be left with open, raw wounds. Awareness of these overwhelmingly painful emotions may lead to an increased risk of suicide. A weekend workshop may introduce the process of therapy, but some provision for ongoing and follow-up care is necessary for clients with clinical issues.

Avoid Being Exploited

If you feel at all exploited in a therapy situation, you must take immediate action. What is exploitation? Keep in mind that the purpose of the therapy is to meet the client's goals and needs. The focus of the work should consistently and unwaveringly be on the client's needs. When the focus of the work shifts toward meeting the therapist's needs, the risk of exploitation is high. If the therapist talks about her own problems, the focus cannot be on her client.

If at anytime you feel exploited, voice your concerns to your therapist. She should respond actively by clarifying perspectives and addressing concerns with necessary changes. If she does not actively respond to concerns, seek consultation. Evaluate the need for changing therapists or treatment approaches.

Although it is shameful, sexual exploitation does occur in the therapy office. Because of transference feelings, clients are vulnerable to becoming emotionally dependent on the therapist. When a therapist acts on sexual impulses with a client, it is the emotional equivalent of incest. In many cases, sexual exploitation of a therapy client is illegal and carries serious penalties. If your therapist approaches you sexually, stop therapy and seek consultation. In addition, if you have sexual impulses toward your therapist, discuss them, do not act on them. Sexual behavior has no place in psychotherapy. It should involve essentially no physical contact.

Beware of therapies that demand payment in advance or fees that are unrealistically high. If you believe that you are being financially exploited by your therapist, discuss the difficulty. Review fee structures that are standard in your area. Be honest in all your communications with insurance companies. Do not agree to falsify information to third-party payers. Check that dates billed match dates of attendance on all insurance forms. If you need treatment and are unable to pay, a therapist can assist you in accessing mental health resources in your area.

Avoid Cults

A cult is a religious group with a common set of devotional practices. Often, members have been brainwashed or coerced into following an ideology. Members of cults are influenced by techniques of mind control and manipulation of thoughts. They are forced to adopt the values and ideas of the group, or they are rejected from the group. Group members in a cult are highly dependent emotionally, and at times, physically dependent on the group to meet their needs.

Above all, a therapy must leave you a free thinker. A cult involves brainwashing. You must follow the thinking of the group in order to belong to it. Therapy does not require any religious observation or devotional practice. You can discuss new perspectives with your therapist, but the choice about how to think, feel, and act is ultimately yours.

This may come as a disappointment to some people. Clients are surprisingly too willing to turn over decision making to the therapist. They ask: "What should I do about the job?" "How should I feel toward my parents?" "Wouldn't you be angry?" Even if this level of dependence were possible, would you really want it? Why let someone else define your experience? Can they really do a better job than you? Don't you offer your own unique spin?

You must evaluate the therapy process actively. Any form of therapy should be open to discussion with providers and significant others. Ask people who know about therapy, share experiences, and read about the process. Consult with another provider.

CHAPTER 13

So You're Cured, or At Least Discharged?

By nature, human beings are always evolving. We are a work in progress. Once you have learned a new way of thinking in therapy, that skill will always be a part of your coping strategies. Having learned the process, you can use it anywhere, anytime, for years. Clients will experience varying degrees of relief in therapy. Some symptoms may be eliminated, others only controlled. At some point, you will decide to end formal meetings and discontinue the work in-session. The experiences of therapy can persist, as you apply what you have learned in real life, use your understanding, and continue to make changes in behavioral responses. The gains belong to you. You will take them with you to use long after formal meetings have ended.

In many therapies, the decision to stop is a mutual one, where the therapist and the client agree that a natural stopping point has been reached. In other situations, ending treatment may be imposed because of a lack of insurance reimbursement or changes in the availability of the therapist.

Some treatment settings use students to provide therapy, and when the training period is over, the client may need to change to another therapist. If the therapy ends for reasons other than the client's desire, the impact of the termination will be different.

When the decision to stop is a mutual one, ending can be used to examine progress. Areas for future work might be identified, but plans to address these issues will rest with the client. If therapy termination is because of the situation or the therapist, the client may feel abandoned. Feelings of anger and a lack of trust might arise.

Termination

The decision to end treatment should never be made lightly. If you are thinking of leaving treatment, it is important to discuss this with your therapist. Some clients consider abruptly terminating treatment, particularly when feelings in therapy become uncomfortable. The client may be reluctant to discuss these thoughts with the therapist. Ending is an opportunity to consider how far the client has come toward meeting their goals. Once the topic of ending treatment comes up, it is not unusual to see a recurrence of symptoms that initially brought the client into treatment. This is generally an anxiety response and is temporary. The decision to stop treatment should not necessarily be postponed if this happens, rather, the client should begin to rely on his own resources to resolve unwanted symptoms. The therapist should continue to support the client's autonomy and progress toward discharge. A date should be made for a final meeting.

Many people have a brief period of treatment, then complete termination successfully. The client and the therapist may wish to leave open the option to return to treatment in the future. Once the relationship of therapist to client is established, this is a lifelong arrangement. This means that in order to uphold the ethical requirements to avoid dual relationships, once termination occurs, the structure of the relationship cannot change. Because the option to return to treatment exists, a social relationship cannot occur after termination. There is really no time limit to the therapist-client contract. It is not uncommon to hear from a client again, many years after treatment has ended.

The Consolidation Phase

Consolidation begins to occur with the decision to terminate. The process that goes on after the formal treatment meetings end involves incorporation of new ways of thinking and acting, as well as integration of insights. The client is changed because of the therapeutic interaction. What remains and what is discarded depends on the client's utilization of information and awareness achieved in treatment. In beginning to rely solely on their own judgment and perceptions, clients may be anxious, but after a prolonged treatment, the therapist's perspective becomes available as introject within the person. The effects of extended treatment tend to be relatively permanent because the therapy was, in essence, also a real experience in the client's mental history.

Once the decision to end treatment is accepted, regular meetings will be suspended. Many clients experience feelings of loss over no longer having uninterrupted periods of supportive attention. There is a loss of relationship that involved trust and confidence. However, the client takes with him an introject or incorporated object representation of the therapist. There is a new voice in the client's head that asks "How does that feel" or counteracts other critical thoughts. The client takes with him a memory of a trusting, adequate relationship that valued him for who he is. The client has had the experience of revealing aspects of himself that were previously unacceptable, and having the therapist accept those aspects with a balanced neutrality. These hidden, shameful awarenesses no longer cause such distress and can be acknowledged and then dismissed. Many clients leave therapy with a stronger sense of identity from having examined the various aspects of self. The therapy experience is validating and increases self-esteem.

It is not unusual to have a transient return of symptoms as psychotherapy ends. This may be related to anxiety about stopping treatment, and an unconscious communication to the therapist that they are still needed and valued. The separation at the end of treatment is not unlike other developmental separations. There may be some distress, but these feelings should not stop forward progress. The interruption of the relationship offers the opportunity for an experience of mastery over the separation process.

Some clients may wish to terminate treatment gradually, scheduling progressively longer intervals between appointments. These final appointments can serve a supportive purpose and allow for an extended appraisal about the decision to interrupt treatment.

The therapeutic contract extends for life, and, in fact, into death. It is potentially damaging to the client, if after formal treatment ends, a different type of relationship is attempted. The client has been in a position of vulnerability, and the risk of the therapist exploiting lingering feelings is high. Be forewarned that if a new type of relationship, such as friendship, is attempted, the responsibility to protect the client from harm and exploitation rests solely with the practitioner. In order not to commit an ethical violation, dual relationships are to be avoided at all costs.

Returning to Treatment

Clients will often contact a therapist for a consultation years after extended treatment has ended. It is not unusual for a therapist in practice in the same area to hear from a client fif-

teen years later. It is a good idea to clarify options for returning to treatment with the therapist prior to ending treatment.
Most therapists will remain available to the client as needed.

Some clients may wish to touch base with the therapist
periodically. Although the process of active psychotherapy
may not be possible with intermittent contact, these meetings
may serve several purposes. The therapist and the impact of
the therapy remain an active part of the client's mental life.
There may be a feeling of reassurance at having the therapist
available for consultation. Although contact may be infrequent, the client may still use the therapist as an image of
mental support. There may be a sense that somewhere in the
world there is someone who understands and is concerned
about your well-being.

It may be reassuring to know that if symptoms reappear,
it is possible to restart active work in psychotherapy. It may
be that traumatic events later in life reactivate old issues and
prompt a return to the therapy process. In addition, it may be
natural to use the process of psychotherapy, so beneficial in
the past, to assist in meeting developmental challenges. For
example, someone who had a positive experience with therapy in their young-adult years may return to therapy to address empty nest feelings, or in later years to deal with feelings
about aging. In addition, it may be that at one point in life, an
issue appears to be resolved to satisfaction. For example, anxieties about abandonment, which linger from the adolescent
years, seem resolved after therapy in the twenties. However,
reaching a new developmental phase, such as the death of
one's parents, may cause these issues to resurface. In this new
phase of life, issues can be reexamined and understood at a
deeper level, with the wisdom of maturity and experience.

CHAPTER 14

Resources

Information and Support

When we are struggling with an emotional or psychological challenge, there may be a natural tendency to seek out others who may have information about our interests. Learning from others about emotional difficulty can be valuable in many ways. It can help you decide on a course of action or treatment, and may help soften negative opinions you might have about mental illness. Understanding, through information, may decrease shame and guilt. Finding others with common concerns will also decrease a sense of isolation.

Organizations

Here are some national organizations that provide support and information related to mental health issues. Some of these groups also have local chapters, which will be listed in the blue or white pages of your phone book. If you are searching for answers or resources, don't hesitate to call or write these organizations. In addition, many have a page on the Internet and can be accessed digitally.

Al-Anon Family Groups
National Public Information
P.O. Box 5433, Station J
Ottawa, Ontario, K2A 3Y6
Canada
(613) 722-1830
Twelve-step fellowship programs for family members and
loved ones of clients with addictions.

Alcoholics Anonymous
475 Riverside Dr.
New York, NY 10163
(212) 870-3400
Twelve-step fellowship programs for people with a desire to
achieve sobriety from alcohol.

Alzheimer's Association
919 N. Michigan Ave., Suite 1000
Chicago, IL 60611
(312) 335-8700
1-800-272-3900
Information clearinghouse for material related to Alzheimer's
Disease.

American Academy of Pediatrics
141 Northwest Point Blvd.
Box 927
Elk Grove, IL 60609-0927
1-800-433-9016
Professional organization for pediatricians. Supports
exchange of information and research findings.

American Anorexia and Bulimia Association
293 Central Park West, Suite 1R
New York, NY 10024

(212) 501-8351
Information clearinghouse for material related to eating
disorders.

American Association of Children's Residential Centers
1021 Prince St.
Alexandria, VA 22314-2971
Professional organization for clinicians involved in residential
treatment for children.

American Association for Marriage and Family Therapy
1100 17th St., NW, 10th Fl.
Washington, DC 20036
Professional organization for marital and family therapists.
Sponsors educational programs and professional development.

American Association of Retired Persons (AARP)
601 E St., NW
Washington, DC 20049
(202) 434-2227
Organization for adults fifty-five and older. Provides
information, sponsors consumer advocacy, and support
for clients.

American Counseling Association
5999 Stevenson Ave.
Alexandria, VA 22304-3300
Professional organization for counselors.

American Hospital Association
840 North Lake Shore Dr.
Chicago, IL 60611
(312) 280-6000
Focuses on issues related to standards for hospital
administration.

American Nurses Association
600 Maryland Ave., SW, Suite 100 West
Washington, DC 20024
(202) 554-4444
Professional organization for nurses.

American Orthopsychiatric Association
1370 Lamberton Dr.
Silver Springs, MD 20902
Organization dedicated to an interdisciplinary approach to individual and societal issues.

American Psychiatric Association
1400 K St., NW
Washington, DC 20005
(202) 682-6000
National organization for psychiatrists. Facilitates exchange of information and research, promotes public interest, governs education, and ethical standards.

American Psychoanalytic Association
309 East 49th St.
New York, NY 10017
(212) 750-0450
Fax (212) 593-0571
National organization of psychoanalysts. Facilitates exchange of information and training of psychoanalysts. Good resource of information about treatment and for listing of available clinicians.

American Psychological Association
750 1st St., NE
Washington, DC 20002
(202) 336-5500
National professional organization for psychologists. Provides

for exchange of professional information and research; facilitates public mental health interests; promotes education in psychology; and governs the practice of psychology by establishing ethical standards.

American Psychological Society
1010 Vermont Ave., NW, Suite 1100
Washington, DC 20005-4907
Professional interest group for psychologists.

Anxiety Disorder Association of America
6000 Executive Blvd.
Rockville, MD 20852
(301) 231-9350
Information clearinghouse for material relating to anxiety disorders.

Association for the Advancement of Behavior Therapy
305 7th Ave., Suite 16A
New York, NY 10001
(212) 647-1890
Interest group that promotes advances in behavior therapy.

CPI (National Crisis Prevention Institute, Inc.)
3315-KN 124th St.
Brookfield, WI 53005
(414) 783-5787
Organization designed to prevent and manage crises in children.

Child Welfare League of America
440 First St., NW, Suite 310
Washington, DC 20001-2085
(202) 638-2952

Dedicated to protecting the rights of children. Provides advocacy and direct support for children.

Clearinghouse on Child Abuse and Neglect Information
P.O. Box 1182
Washington, DC 20013
(703) 385-7565
Information clearinghouse.

Family Service of America
1319 F St., NW, Suite 204
Washington, DC 20004
Non-profit organization dedicated to fostering family functioning. Provides education and social services.

Gerontological Society of America
1275 K St., NW, Suite 350
Washington, DC 20005-4006
(202) 842-1275
Professional organization and information clearinghouse.

Incest Survivors Anonymous
P.O. Box 1745
Long Beach, CA 90807-7245
(310) 428-5599

Lithium Information Center
OCD Information Center
The Dean Foundation for Health, Research, and Education
8000 Excelsior Dr., Suite 302
Madison, WI 53717-1914
(608) 836-8070
Information clearinghouse.

National Alliance for the Mentally Ill (NAMI)
200 North Glebe Rd., Suite 1015
Arlington, VA 22203-3754
(702) 524-7600
Helpline: 1-800-950-6264
Advocacy and support group for family members of clients
with mental illness. Offers support-group meetings,
information about illness and treatment, action-group lobbies
for legislative change at community and national levels. Also
has an extensive library of information available at a low cost,
including pamphlets, books, audiotapes, and videos.

National Anxiety Foundation
3135 Custer Dr.
Lexington, KY 40517
(606) 272-7166
Information clearinghouse related to anxiety.

National Association of Home Care
205 C St., NE
Washington, DC 20002
(202) 547-7424
Information and referral related to home care issues.

National Association of Psychiatric Survivors
P.O. Box 618
Sioux Falls, SD 57101-0618
(605) 334-4067
Support group for clients with mental health issues.

National Association of Social Workers
750 1st St., NE
Washington, DC 20001
Professional organization for social workers.

National Council on Alcoholism, Inc.
12 W 21st St.
New York, NY 10010
(212) 206-6770
Information clearinghouse for material about alcoholism.
Sponsors education and research programs.

National Clearinghouse for Alcohol and Drug Information
P.O. Box 2345
Rockville, MD 20847-2345
1-800-628-1696
Informational resources.

National Depressive and Manic Depressive Association
730 North Franklin St., Suite 501
Chicago, IL 60610
Information related to bipolar and unipolar depressions.

National Foundation for Depressive illness
P.O. Box 2257
New York, NY 10116
Information clearinghouse.

National Institute on Aging
Public Information Office
Federal Building, Room 5C27, Building 31
9000 Rockville Pl.
Bethesda, MD 20892
(301) 496-1752
Sponsors research and advocacy efforts for older adults.

National Institute of Mental Health (NIMH)
Room 7C-02
5600 Fishers Ln.

Rockville, MD 20857
(301) 443-4513
Part of Health and Human Services, National Institutes of
Health. Clearinghouse for information and research activities
in the United States. Provides government grants and
financial assistance to research efforts. Distributes
information on etiology and treatment of mental health
difficulties.

National Mental Health Association
1021 Prince St.
Alexandria, VA 22314
Advocacy group. Professional organization for mental health
providers.

National Mental Health Consumers Association
P.O. Box 1166
Madison, WI 53701
Support and advocacy for clients with mental health issues.

National Mental Health Consumers Self-Help Clearinghouse
c/o Community Support Programs of the Center for Mental
Health Services, Substance Abuse and Mental Health Services
Administration
211 Chestnut St., Suite 1000
Philadelphia, PA 19107
1-800-553-4539

Recovery, Inc.
802 North Dearborn St.
Chicago, IL 60610
(312) 337-5661
Support groups for clients with mental health issues.

The Obsessive-Compulsive Foundation
P.O. Box 70
Milford, CT 06460-0070
1-800-639-7462
Informatiocn and referral related to Obsessive-Compulsive
Disorder.

Overeaters Anonymous
6075 Zenith Court, Northeast
Rio Ranchero, NM 87124-6424
(505) 891-2664
Support group for clients with overeating behaviors.

Schizophrenics Anonymous
1209 California Rd.
Eastchester, NY 10709
(914) 337-2252
Support group for clients with schizophrenia.

Society for Traumatic Stress Studies
435 North Michigan Ave., Suite 171
Chicago, IL 60611-4067
(312) 644-0828
Conducts research and provides educational programs on
Traumatic Stress Disorders.

State and Local Organizations

Look in the front of your phone book to identify local resources that may be useful. Don't hesitate to call, and ask
about available services. Each state has a psychological association and a psychiatric association. In addition, there may be
local groups of clinicians or self-help groups in larger cities.

Internet and Websites

The Internet is full of information about mental health issues. The World Wide Web has created a communications explosion that allows us to share health-related discoveries almost instantly. With the coming of the electronic/digital communication age, researchers in remote areas can share findings immediately. This allows a global group-think as never before possible, dedicated to the search for answers to health-related problems.

Many people have personal computers that facilitate access to the Internet. If you do not have your own personal computer, there are other ways to connect with the information highway. Because of the importance of the Internet in research, your local library may have computers that have Internet capability for your use. Coffeehouses with Internet access are becoming increasingly popular. These *cybercafes* allow you to pay a small fee to use their computer connections. You can surf the Net while sipping a latte. In addition, there are franchises of commercial office sites, such as Kinko's, which offer computer services. For a fee, you can use their computers to link up with information on the Web. Some people are choosing to bypass the computer altogether and access the internet with Web-TV. These systems allow you, for several hundred dollars, to surf the Net via your television. Anyone can log on. Don't let the mechanics interfere with getting the information.

Information about mental health is available at thousands of sites! In addition to commercial sites and consumer-interest pages, there is information from government sources, such as the National Institutes of Health or the Center for Disease Control. Look for university home pages to obtain information about research and faculty activities. Bulletin boards can offer lively discussion groups. Perhaps the best way to find these sites is to use a search engine (Yahoo, Netscape, Lycos) with key words: mental health, psychology, or psychotherapy. There are many sites devoted to specific diagnostic issues, such as eating disorders, substance-abuse recovery, obsessive-compulsive disorder, depression, dementia, and personality disorders. There are sites that provide information about clinicians in your area, as well as link you with other interesting surfers.

It is important that you carefully evaluate any information found on the World Wide Web. The Internet is truly a *surfer beware* environment. There are no regulations to protect readers. When a mental health professional publishes an article, there are ethical guidelines that protect the reader from false information or false credentials. On the Web, anyone can write anything. If someone discovers that standing on your head three times a day cures depression, they can put this information out on a Web page or bulletin board. They may not have done any clinical studies, and there may be no empirical evidence to support their claims. On the Web there is the suspension of disbelief. Anyone can say they are a therapist; you cannot see their license to practice through a modem. However, not everyone on the Internet is a fake. Many credible authors and professionals make valuable, accurate information available over the Web. The Internet can be a spectacular networking method that is global and instantaneous.

Some sites offer diagnostic surveys that you can complete to determine if you meet criteria for specific disorders, such as depression or anxiety. These surveys may come from accepted tools, such as the Beck Depression Inventory, which is easy to self-administer and score. However, many of these tools can be likened to surveys found in magazines. Some have clinical relevance, others are purely for entertainment. When evaluating a specific disorder, it is important to consult with a qualified clinician if concerns persist.

Several Websites currently offer advice services. Others

even suggest they are offering psychotherapy. Others provide chat rooms for discussing personal concerns. The Internet does not guarantee privacy, even in a chat room. It also does not guarantee that the person dispensing advice is qualified. Some of these sites appear to be offered by clinicians with acceptable credentials. However, again, there is no protection for the consumer against people who may fake being a therapist simply for the purposes of entertainment.

Although I am wary of support services offered on-line, I have also seen clients benefit significantly from these interactions. In one case, I was seeing a woman whose family objected to her taking time away from child care to physically attend a support group. She found a chat room on-line that was devoted to issues similar to her own and was able to interact with these people without leaving the comfort of her home—and without raising concerns from her family. The Internet can link you with information and help you network with others who have similar interests. However, it cannot substitute for a clinical evaluation or professional treatment.

In addition, most professional organizations are establishing an Internet presence. These pages offer networking opportunities for clients, as well as clinicians. Many professional journals are available at these sites.

Here are some Web addresses to get you started:
Http://www.apsa. org
  American Psychoanalytic Association
Http://www.apa.org
  American Psychological Association
Http://www.mentalhealth.org
  The National Mental Health Services Knowledge
  Exchange Network, by U.S. Department of
  Human Services
Http://www.chmc.com
  Mental Health Net

Http://www.counseling.org
American Counseling Association

Publications

Commercial and professional publications offer a wealth of information about psychology and mental health issues. Magazines frequently carry articles about emotional difficulties. The psychology and self-help sections in the bookstore are overflowing with information and advice. Newspapers often run segments with articles about mental health, which are contributed by local psychotherapists. This information can help you become an educated consumer, as well as learn what others are saying. However, as with the Internet, you must critically evaluate what is being said. Assess the author's credentials to understand the perspectives of the article or book. Discuss the perspectives with others to learn what supports the views that are offered. Is there research to back up his findings? Does your personal experience match or contradict the author's perspectives? Keep an open mind when you are reading, but be critical as you evaluate various perspectives.

Professional publications provide in-depth information but may be too technical for some people. When reading information designed for professionals, you must be careful not to misinterpret clinical terms. Professionals often write for each other using vocabulary that is shorthand and can be easily misunderstood. For example, when reading the descriptions of personality disorders in *DSM,* you might come across such terms as *mood swings* or *identity confusion.* Many people might say, "I have those symptoms!" However, what is referred to here is beyond ordinary fluctuations in mood or normal questions about identity and self-concept. Clinicians are trained to distinguish between what is ordinary and what is a clinical symptom. The terms used in describing these disorders have specific meanings. If you are reading material intended for a professional audience, you may wish to discuss it with a professional to better understand how, or even if, it applies to you.

Broadcast Media

Commercial broadcasts devote a great deal of attention to psychological disorders and treatment. Often, discoveries about clinical conditions and treatments are covered by local and prime-time news shows. Documentaries, special-interest segments, and stories that cover professional journals can offer a valuable source of information, particularly about the latest research. A number of news programs covers what is being published in journals such as the *New England Journal of Medicine* and the *Journal of the American Medical Association*; these programs translate these stories for the general public. In addition, commercial media regularly feature information about developments in health-care policy and research. Broadcast and printed media frequently remind us that there are ways to improve our health. More than ever, as a public, we are aware of disorders, treatments, and diagnostic options.

Films and Videos

Since ancient Rome and Greece, we have illustrated the dramas and comedies of life on the stage. This tradition continues with the film industry. Today, we can learn about human experience through the cinema. A picture is truly worth a thousand words. Hollywood has long been fascinated with psychological conflict. Many specific disorders have been portrayed on the big screen. In addition, there are many professionally prepared films about treatment, development, and disorders. Check local university libraries for lending and viewing policies. Psychological conflicts and dramas are documented in truth and in fiction on film. A wealth of information about psychological conditions awaits the dedicated move watcher. Some films will take liberties with a story and dramatize a situation for effect. Others offer a realistic portrayal of a clinical condition and the recovery process. At the very least, films can stimulate a discussion about important personal or societal mental health issues. So fire up your membership card, and search for these exciting portrayals! (These are just a few suggestions; undoubtedly, you will be able to add many more to the list.

Annie Hall

Woody Allen has given us an education in psychotherapy. He shows us how the process of exploration works and helps us laugh at our neuroses.

Birdy

This is a film that illustrates a client with a delusional disorder. After experiencing the trauma of war, the client develops the belief that he is a bird. This is an interesting illustration of a break from reality, as well as a poignant exploration of friendship.

Clean and Sober This is a film about substance dependence and recovery. It offers the story of several people in the early stages of recovery from addiction. The film shows an AA meeting and portrays the relationship between sponsor and member. The story illustrates many common issues encountered in the recovery process, including withdrawal, family communication, and coping with impulses to use.

Fatal Attraction Glenn Close portrays a classic example of a young woman with a borderline personality disorder—a textbook example of the unstable traits in this erratic character disorder.

The Fisher King This film provides an illustration of an atypical posttraumatic stress disorder. Robin Williams plays a widower who is psychotic with grief. This film offers a glimpse of what the world is like for someone who is psychotic (or out of touch with reality). One scene illustrates how we might begin to understand seemingly inexplicable behavior. Robin Williams is talking to someone on the street, then suddenly begins to scream and run away. At first this seems bizarre, but when seen from his altered perspective, there is a fire-breathing dragon chasing him, reigning terror! This scene can illustrate that when perspective is understood, most behavior will make some sense.

Frances This is the story of a young woman wrongly confined to a mental institution.

I Never Promised You a Rose Garden This story of a woman with schizophrenia shows a positive relationship with a therapist.

Nuts This brilliant film illustrates several important legal issues in mental health, including the right to stand trial and the insanity defense. It offers an explanation of how we define mental illness, and the hypocrisy of what we call *normal*.

One Flew Over the Cuckoo's Nest A classic film about the structure and function of the psychiatric system, as well as a humorous exploration of psychological difficulties. It illustrates the effects of the prefrontal lobotomy and created the timeless image of Nurse Rachet.

Ordinary People This is an excellent film that explores family dynamics, depression, suicide, and provides a beautiful illustration of the therapeutic relationship. It is the story of depression in a family as a result of the death of a child. Judd Hirsch portrays a compassionate, skilled clinician. One caveat with the film: I am wary of the characterization of the relationship between client and therapist as a friendship. There are distinct differences between social and therapeutic relationships.

The Prince of Tides This horrifying film sends shivers down the spine of any ethical therapist! It contains so many ethical violations that it is a frightening model to put forth to the public. First, the therapist begins to do therapy with her patient's brother. This is a dual relationship that the client did not consent to. The therapist violates client confidentiality. She doesn't charge for her service. And most horrifying, she sleeps with her client. The scenes portrayed in this movie parallel some clients' fantasies about what the therapy relationship will be like—no doubt this contributes to the film's popularity. But fantasies about having a sexual relationship or about being held while weeping need to be discussed, not acted on. This film is a good example of "what to avoid" in therapy.

Regarding Henry This is an excellent example of a client with a brain injury. It illustrates the rehabilitative process. Although the ultimate impact of a brain injury is somewhat idealistic, this story of recovery is loosely accurate.

The Snake Pit This classic film from the 1950s stars Olivia deHavilland as a young woman with psychotic depression. This film takes you inside the world of the state mental institution and allows you to see inside the closed wards and examples of a variety of diagnoses, as well as institutional functioning. This film illustrates the process of the talking cure and gives a nice example of a patient-therapist relationship.

Stuart Saves His Family This is a delightful satire of the self-help movement and family dysfunction. This film manages to capture the tenets of twelve-step programs and takes a satirical look at family relationships.

Sweetie This film may be hard to find, but it is worth watching. It is a portrait of a family that struggles with chronic mental illness. Sweetie has bipolar disorder and does an accurate job of illustrating symptoms. Life for clients with bipolar disorder can unfortunately get as out of control as it does in this movie. A must-see for all students of abnormal psychology!

The Three Faces of Eve This is a classic story based on a true case. This film offers a realistic portrayal of a young woman with multiple personalities. In the Hollywood version there are three Eves: Eve White, Eve Black, and Jane. In reality, there were many more segments of Eve's personality.

Titticutt Follies: The Documentary This film is hard to come by. It was not originally released to the general public and may still only be available to students and professionals. It is the story of several patients at the Bridgewater State Mental Hospital as they prepare and present a stage show for entertainment and alleged therapeutic purposes. It is a realistic documentation of actual conditions in a mental institution in upstate Massachusetts, circa 1960.

Twelve Monkeys This popular film portrays life in a mental hospital in a surreal fashion. It is not a realistic portrayal of life in a psychiatric hospital today. Perhaps some institutions in the past resemble where Brad Pitt is hospitalized, but in reality, this dramatization was filmed in an old prison for effect. Hospitals are extremely conscious of client's rights and every attempt to maintain a humane social environment is made. In this film, Pitt plays someone diagnosed with schizophrenia. In reality, his disorder more closely resembles someone with a bipolar disorder or delusional disorder. He does not exhibit the disorganization that is characteristic of schizophrenia but does offer a brilliant look into the world of delusions, and calls us to listen closely to the rantings of madmen!

What About Bob This is your therapist's worst nightmare: a client who relentlessly invades the therapist's private life. See this one for its absurd comedic value.

For more information see *Psychiatry and the Cinema* by Gabbard and Gabbard, University of Chicago Press, 1987.

In addition, many films developed for use by clinicians are also available. Two examples include:

Breaking the Silence, available from the American Psychiatric Association, 1-800-366-8455. A film about sexual abuse and children, it focuses on the resolution of issues in treatment and the prevention of abuse.

Broken Minds, available from the American Psychiatric Association, 1-800-366-8455. An informative piece about the history of schizophrenia and current treatment.

The best way to obtain films such as these is with the assistance of your local community or university library.

CHAPTER 15

Becoming a Psychotherapist

S ome of you may be reading this because you are interested in becoming a psychotherapist. Congratulations on choosing one of the most fascinating and rewarding areas of study and practice. Every day presents something new. When you work with people, no two days are ever the same. I hope you are privileged to interact with clients from all walks of life, a wide variety of cultural backgrounds, and with all manner of ego strengths and limitations. As the Chinese proverb says, "May you live in interesting times." I might add, "and with interesting people."

Many of us decide to become psychotherapists because we have seen firsthand the positive effects of treatment. Perhaps we have watched a skilled clinician work with family or friends. Sometimes, we have been in therapy ourselves. Somewhere we discovered that psychotherapy can produce positive results, and we decide to share this discovery with others.

There are many motivations for becoming a psychotherapist. Often, clinicians begin their work in the healing arts that target the physical body, such as medicine or nursing. Seeing the impact of the mind on physical illness, we begin to study psychology and adaptation. Often potential clinicians have had a helping role in their families while growing up. When this is the case, the role of therapist may come naturally.

It is often said that we become psychotherapists in order to heal our own emotional and psychological wounds. Even though this has been said in jest, it is true that curiosity about our own functioning leads us to further study the mind. The decision to become a therapist may be motivated by esteem needs, and the need for prestige. Therapists are often given significant power in today's society, even to the extent of being overvalued. The title *doctor* carries with it recognition of a level of expertise in understanding the mind. Like members of the clergy, many people imagine that therapists have special abilities. It may be disappointing to learn that therapists are ordinary people with ordinary problems.

Perhaps the most often cited reason for wanting to become a psychotherapist is, "I want to help people." And certainly, that is part of why we all become psychotherapists. It is gratifying to be able to facilitate someone's development, or to support problem-solving efforts. We are reaffirmed as human beings when our interactions lead to positive outcomes and optimal adaptation.

Helping is an admirable quality, but it is not enough to sustain a career. If you have a tendency to be codependent or to focus on others rather than attending to yourself, you may not be able to be effective as a therapist. Martyrs do not make good therapists. Altruism is a rare quality. But the practice of therapy is a vocation, not charity. The client must, by definition, put more effort into change than the therapist. Clients who overcome difficulties devote significant energy to introspection, self-observation, and conscious behavioral choices. Change cannot be created with the therapist's energy alone. The energy for the process and the desire for change must come from the client.

If you are considering becoming a therapist, it is important to discover what is motivating that choice. The first part of your journey must involve self-exploration and developing an understanding of what makes you want to pursue this career path. It is important to know your own motivations to minimize the impact these forces will have on your work. If you have a strong hidden agenda, clients will not be free to work in the direction and process that is uniquely theirs. For example, if your desire to become a therapist is motivated primarily by a need to help people get well, then it may be difficult for you to work with clients who are experiencing exacerbation of symptoms. Professional therapists have a commitment to work with clients who are doing well *and* those who are not doing well. If you are motivated by prestige, it may be difficult when clients devalue the contributions of mental health disciplines.

It is important to approach becoming a therapist with motivation sufficient to sustain rigorous years of study. For example, you may be interested in helping and learning about the processes of the mind, and you may want a responsible, challenging career. When a number of factors support the motivation to become a therapist, the energy needed to pursue that path is more likely to be consistently available. The therapist's personal agenda is less likely to be played out in work with clients.

Psychotherapy should be viewed as a skill. It is one form of intervention. It is a complex intervention guided by a large body of knowledge, and takes effort and discipline to learn. Many forms of helping relationships exist. Deciding to become a therapist rather than some other form of helper requires a dedication to formal study, clinical practice, and personal development.

A genuine interest in the human condition is a necessary prerequisite for study of the mind. If you are curious about the human experience, it will be easier to survive the rigors of academic preparation necessary to practice psychotherapy. Although the energy needed to work with people may come easily, the discipline needed to complete doctoral-level training may not.

Do not become a therapist for the money. The mental health system is depleted of resources. If you think you will get rich practicing psychotherapy, think again. Many years before the health-care crisis, Freida Frohm-Reichman recommended that therapists have another source of income to facilitate the private practice of psychotherapy. Through positions in academia, hospitals, or consulting firms, therapists can be free from the burden of earning a living from private psychotherapy clients. This recommendation is an attempt to separate financial from treatment concerns in psychotherapy. The therapist can be freer to make decisions about fees based on the clinical aspects of the case rather than his own financial need.

Do become a psychotherapist if you are genuinely interested in people. If you are willing to work hard, both in formal training and in self-exploration, you may be a successful candidate for the field. There are a number of benefits to considering a career as a psychotherapist. There is a great deal of autonomy in private practice. The work is always varied, continuously new, and challenging. The relationships with clients and colleagues are satisfying and frequently stimulate ongoing personal growth. If you are interested in human nature and see participation in study and relationships as a way to grow—for yourself and others—you may be well suited to a career in counseling. Benefits must not be only one-sided. You are entitled to a fulfilling career that inadvertently—perhaps incidentally—will be helpful to others.

Education

If you are interested in becoming a psychotherapist, you must study everything! Try to get exposure to as many perspectives as possible. Don't discount a theory until you have studied and evaluated it closely. Read everything! Study different disciplines, including history, religion, society, biology, and philosophy. A broad education is an important way to develop critical-thinking skills and autonomous reasoning. Becoming a psychotherapist involves graduate education, then licensure in the practice of a profession. Advanced education must focus on theories of human functioning and include perspectives on physiology, behavior, personality, and psychology. Give balanced attention to each theoretical perspective. A solid, liberal arts, or applied-science education and some experience working in the field is desirable.

Undergraduate preparation for becoming a therapist may include a broad liberal arts education, or any area of humanities, business, or sciences. A bachelor's degree in any area of study may be useful to prepare a student for advanced graduate study. Some graduate programs prefer that candidates have a background in psychology or mental health. Other programs prefer non-psychology backgrounds, such as business, social work, history, nursing, or fine arts. Undergraduate education should prepare the student for advanced study. The process of earning a bachelor's degree develops character and personality, as well as disciplined study habits.

In general, the practice of psychotherapy requires a graduate education. Beyond a basic level of study, as a society we agree that people who practice therapy should have advanced training. Getting into graduate school is a challenge. Entrance exams that tap necessary language, math, and reasoning skills are usually required. Preparation for these should be long term. Most programs ask for Graduate Record Exams or Miller analogies. Many people are not accepted into graduate study programs with the first year of applications. Do not let this discourage you. Apply again the next year. Schools consider diligence and persistence when evaluating academic goals. Graduate study can be undertaken in a number of different disciplines in order to prepare the therapist to offer consultation.

The science of medicine offers preparation to practice therapy in psychiatric training programs. If you are interested in physiological perspectives and are capable of rigorous academic work, in order to become a psychiatrist you must complete four years of medical school. After obtaining this doctorate, three or four years of residency training in psychiatry are necessary. The focus of medical school curriculum and residency training should offer the therapist in-depth understanding of biological, pharmacological, and psychological functioning. Increasingly, medical training comes from a holistic perspective. When this is combined with a residency that teaches the practice of psychotherapy, the result can be a highly skilled clinician.

You may decide that you prefer graduate education in psychology as preparation for practice. The minimum requirement for becoming a psychologist is a doctorate level of education. The focus of graduate programs in psychology includes intellectual and personality functioning, ethics, theories of the mind and behavior, learning theory, and specialized subjects, such as neurological functioning, clinical psychology, or experimental psychology. Obtaining a doctorate in psychology also involves rigorous study and generally has a research component. In addition to qualifying exams, a dissertation and original research are required.

The discipline of social work offers preparation for practicing psychotherapy. A master's degree in social work, along with licensure, allows you to become a therapist. Graduate social work education focuses on psychosocial systems, as well as individual and family functioning. In the future, the discipline of social work may follow other fields and make a doctorate in social work the standard for entry into practice.

Nursing also offers educational preparation for becoming a therapist. A master's degree in psychiatric or mental health nursing can provide the foundation for practice. Clinical specialists in nursing offer therapy from a number of theoretical perspectives, including nursing theory, psychiatry, and psychology.

Some educators recommend studying everything, then

forgetting it all. This caution is important, particularly for beginning clinicians. Students of psychotherapy tend to cling to their theories, relating every occurrence to theories studied in books. The best preparation for the practice of psychotherapy is a course of study that leaves a number of ideas available to the clinician as she focuses efforts on listening to the client. For example, rather than attempting to fit what the client says into a Freudian model, the therapist who studies Freud and then forgets him will be able to listen closely and spontaneously recognize unconscious conflicts, or the symbolism in dreams.

Experience working in the mental health or a health-care setting is helpful. Many graduate programs expect to see some experience in a clinical setting as a part of the requirements for entrance. At times, candidates may obtain support positions after receiving a bachelor's degree. For example, someone with a bachelor's degree in social work may become a case manager in a community mental health center in order to learn more about individual adaptation and system functioning. Someone applying to medical school might volunteer in a local senior citizen home or emergency room. People with a bachelor's degree in psychology might work as vocational or residential counselors in a mental health setting. Graduate programs consider these experiences as demonstrating sustained interest and personal knowledge of mental health settings.

Clinical Practice

You can learn about the science of therapy in school and books, but the art of therapy must be developed through practice. In addition to formal education, becoming a therapist requires learning specific skills, such as assessment, diagnosis, and intervention. Psychotherapy is taught through a process of supervised practice. At some point you must leave behind the books and theories and be with people. You need to try helping and see what effect your methods have. You can use what you've learned from those who have shared their experiences in literature, but ultimately, you must use yourself to try to affect your clients.

At first, the student of psychotherapy may feel as if she's faking it, just sitting in a chair, looking and sounding like a therapist. I believe this quickly fades as the new therapist becomes absorbed in listening to the client. The student may be surprised to discover that the simple listening that the new therapist offers has a profound therapeutic effect.

Beginning practice may make the student feel anxious. This anxiety can be useful in motivating the new therapist to carefully evaluate the client and any interventions. The new therapist listens closely for data and actively compares what is found with theoretical frameworks.

Perhaps the most important factor in supporting the new therapist in beginning work is the supervising therapist. She is responsible for the student's work. She will assess the client, either in person or through the student's account, and will monitor the progress in therapy. The student and therapist work together to support clinical work. A good supervisor can understand the student's level of ability and offers a perspective of the treatment that is once removed from the therapy session. This allows for a slower examination of the therapy process. Associations to patterns in the treatment can be examined over time to better illuminate dynamic processes between the student and the client.

As you begin to see clients, you will encounter many idiosyncrasies in adaptation. You learn how to describe these symptoms and how they cluster in diagnostic categories. You learn how to differentiate clinical syndromes from life's ups and downs. Then you begin to learn the effects of interventions. You watch others practice and learn what body posture and vocal intonations are helpful to communication. Most therapists discover early on that genuineness is important in establishing therapeutic relationships. The new therapist learns to use his own personality style to be effective. Some therapists use a naturally boisterous disposition to be humorous in therapy. Others are quiet and contemplative by nature and well suited to exploratory approaches.

Through clinical practice the student has the opportunity to try new techniques. With the support of supervision, the new therapist can evaluate interventions and select techniques that may not have been tried. The supervisor can make recommendations based on her own clinical experience, as well as an understanding of the nature of the particular case.

Personal Development

Maturity is a valuable quality in a therapist. The therapist must be trustworthy and responsible. Age does not necessarily correlate with maturity. The development of knowledge must be accompanied by the development of character. Most of the counseling professions require that practitioners show evidence of good character. It is not enough to have book knowledge alone. Advising someone on life and intervening with mental life carries with it a profound responsibility. To practice within ethical guidelines, one must, above all else, do no harm. A therapist must cultivate an attitude of respect that allows individuals to form their own opinions; a therapist must genuinely respect the autonomy of clients.

Experience is the Best Teacher

Meet everyone! Greet each person you encounter as an opportunity for learning. Try to interact with people of all ages; listen for the experiences of the old and the young. Seek opportunities to interact with people who are at all levels of adaptation, both brilliant and challenged. Abraham Maslow broke with the tradition of studying clients with symptoms and difficulties and studied people with optimal adjustment in his book *The Farther Reaches of Human Nature*. Try to hear the original authors of theories whenever possible. Watch the lecture circuit for scheduled appearances. Senior clinicians and theorists frequently appear when they are given special awards. Having opportunities to hear the original author present their own work allows you to give a face to the words on the page, and an emotion to intended ideas.

Try to work with clients with diverse complaints and difficulties. Try not to confine clinical experiences to the same segments of the population, for instance, only children or only high-functioning adults. It is best to work with clients who have a broad range of pathology in order to build diagnostic and assessment skills. Learn how to talk with someone who is hallucinating or confused. Learn how to talk with artists, politicians, bankers, and physicians. Spend time with the chronically mentally ill, the homeless, and the gifted.

Travel. Study culture and ethnicity. Whenever possible, see other parts of the world. Learn how religious and ethnic traditions influence thinking and emotion. Seeing a variety of cultures can increase tolerance for different beliefs, values, and customs. Work with rich, poor, urban, rural, all levels of education, all levels of mental functioning, from comatose clients to high-level achievers. The prospective therapist must have experiences with all these people if he wants to develop an understanding of the human experience. The therapist cannot practice if he has only seen one or two types of people. It is important to have a broad range of interactions and human experiences.

Listening

Above all, the therapist must develop the capacity to listen. This is a crucial quality in a counselor. The ability to listen to others is perhaps as important as any theoretical knowledge that can be acquired in school. Beginning therapists are sometimes more effective than experienced clinicians because they are intent on listening. Theodore Reich, renowned analyst, offers a fabulous book called *Listening with the Third Ear.* This work addresses attending to what the client doesn't say, as well as what may be verbally expressed. For example, if a client talks negatively about a parent, it is certain that there also are positive feelings of equal importance that may not be expressed. The therapist must learn to feel the client's experience through listening and imagining.

Therapists must develop empathy, the ability to put yourself in someone else's shoes, to feel and experience vicariously through their expressions. It is a way of profoundly sharing, of bringing another person into a lived experience. It may sound simple, but learning empathy is more like developing a meditative practice. Most people are so preoccupied with themselves that they are constantly busy reacting to their own perceptions, or gathering information to support their views. It takes practice to suspend your own way of seeing the world and to view it through another person's eyes. The best way to develop empathy is to develop listening skills. Listening involves quieting the self—quieting the usually constant chatter of critiques, judgments, or associations that provide running commentary to life's experiences.

Personal Psychotherapy

Preparation for becoming a therapist should involve a personal psychotherapy. Each of us has unresolved issues and unconscious conflicts. To work with helping others, you must be aware of your own functioning. You must know your strengths and weaknesses. You must learn what blind spots may get in the way of seeing your clients. A personal psychotherapy can help minimize the impact of the therapist's personal conflicts in her work. A personal psychotherapy can be a humbling but rewarding experience. The therapist learns how much courage is necessary to even schedule an appointment with a therapist. Through living the experience of therapy, on the couch, a therapist can experience the process of confronting inner demons and the challenges of behavioral change. The potential therapist also experiences the relief of insight and the healing support of the presence of another.

Working as a Psychotherapist

Providing psychotherapy services can be rewarding and challenging. It can be likened to being a midwife. The therapist facilitates the birth of new abilities, experiences, and characteristics. It is recommended that a given psychotherapist provide no more than twenty hours of therapy in a week. This is, in part, because therapy requires significant energy. The therapist must learn to cultivate their own energy resources in order to sustain the progress of work over time.

It is a privilege to be allowed to share someone's personal journey. As a therapist you participate in intimate relationships of exploration and restoration. Each session brings new understanding and insight. You can witness people change and grow.

Practicing psychotherapy also means you will witness suffering. As clients talk of experiences that are uncomfortable and remember events that were traumatic, the therapist is exposed to aspects of life that are unpleasant. The therapist must find ways to balance the awareness of the negative side of life with life-affirming activities and celebrations of the joys of being human. Being a psychotherapist is challenging, interesting, and rewarding.

Glossary

Acting out—Expressing thoughts, feelings, and conflict through overt behaviors. Behaving it rather than saying it.

Adaptation—The process of coping with human experience. Supports the process of survival.

Affects—Feelings or emotions.

Agoraphobia—Fear of being in places from which escape might be difficult or help unavailable in case of anxiety, embarrassment, or panic attack.

Akathesia—Side effect of phenothiazines. Includes restlessness, urge to pace, or an inability to sit still.

Ambivalence—Simultaneously experiencing two opposite feelings or desires.

Anxiety—A sense of apprehension or fear about what might happen. May be associated with feeling uncertain or helpless. Anxiety is a response to perceived threat, either from within one's own mind or the environment.

Behavioral theory—Uses principles of learning and builds on an understanding of principles of conditioning (operant and classical). Examines the relationship between stimulus, organism, and response. Sees mental life as resulting from rewards in the environment and learning from experiences.

Bioenergetics—Method of working with psychological process through physical expression and movements.

Boundary—Physical and psychological limit that denotes where you end and the world begins, and how closely you will allow others to come.

Catharsis—Release of strong emotions to decrease inner tension.

Cognitive theory—Focuses on thinking as the motivator for feelings and behaviors. Emphasizes current thinking rather than past experiences as determinants of mental life.

Compromise formation—A dynamic way of coping with conflicting forces in the psyche that results in a symptom. A compromise between mental forces that attempts to satisfy various needs and wishes.

Conflict—Two opposing forces in the mind, occurring at the same time. Wanting two different things simultaneously.

Counseling—A paraprofessional service that includes support and advice-giving.

Counseling psychologist—Trained in a Rogerian tradition. Provides services that are based on principles of unconditional positive regard, genuineness, and empathy. Focus of treatment is present.

Defenses—Conscious and unconscious mental mechanisms that arise from the ego, which protect us against anxiety.

Deinstitutionalization—Movement to release client from long-term hospitalization and integrate them within the community.

DSM-IV—*Diagnostic and Statistical Manual of Mental Disorders*, fourth edition, a text that describes official criteria for each diagnosis used in this country.

Ego—The part of the mind that balances the demands of internal psychic forces and the demands of the environment and external reality. Governed by the reality principle. Enables us to cope with id impulses and superego admonitions, as well as negotiate daily life.

Enmeshment—Lack of clear boundaries in any relationship. Too much closeness between members.

Hormone—Chemical released by glands and organs in the body, which travels to other organs and regulates activity.

Id—The part of the mind we were born with. Contains basic drives for hunger, closeness, and anger. It is the "I want it, and I want it now!" part of the personality.

Neuropsychologist—A psychologist who specializes in biological brain functioning and brain behavior relationships.

Primary process thinking—Unconscious, dreamlike id patterns of thought. Thinking is symbolic. No means yes, yes means no. It is not logical. Governed by the pleasure principle.

Projection—Unconscious defense mechanism where characteristics present in the self are attributed to others.

Psychiatrist—Someone who has completed medical school and a three- to four-year postdoctoral residency training program in psychiatry. Once training is complete, this person will become Board-Certified by showing proof of educational preparation, and passing a national competency exam.

Psychoanalysis—Form of treatment that involves making the unconscious conscious and resolving conflicts that originate in early life. Generally involves the client reclining on a couch and meetings that take place four or five times a week for several years. The client studies his mental life, using the technique of free association.

Psychoanalyst—A psychologist or psychiatrist with five to ten years of additional training. Can offer psychoanalysis to clients.

Psychoanalytic—Using the ideas derived from Sigmund Freud's work and incorporating modern perspectives that examine unconscious mental life.

Psychodynamic—A contemporary approach that incorporates the tenets of psychoanalytic theory with modern discoveries about mental functioning. Recognizes unconscious mental life and early experiences but also focuses on situational, cognitive, and interpersonal factors.

Psychologist—Someone with an earned doctorate (Ph.D., or Psy.D., or Ed.D.) in the field of psychology, pre- and postdoctoral supervised practice, who has demonstrated minimal competency for practice by passing state and national exams.

Rolfing—Form of therapy that involves bodywork and physical release of emotions.

Secondary process thinking—Logical, ego thinking; reality-based.

Superego—The part of the mind that contains our ideal images of who we should be. Contains conscience. Tells us when we are doing something right or wrong.

Therapist—A generic term meaning anyone who is legally qualified to provide psychotherapy.

Topographic model—Topographic is referring to maps. This is a map of the mind suggested by Freud, which includes conscious, preconscious, and unconscious functioning.

Transference—A mechanism of projection, or the unconscious ascribing of attributes that belong to others to relationships that are current.

References

Allen, C. *Tea With Demons, A True Story* (New York: Ballantine Books, 1985), p.

Anonymous. *Alcoholics Anonymous,* 3rd ed. (World Wide Services, Inc., New York 1976).

Axline, V. M. *Dibs in Search of Self* (New York: Ballantine Books, 1964).

Basch, M. F. *Doing Psychotherapy* (New York: Basic Books, Publishers Inc, 1980).

Berger, L. S. *Substance Abuse as Symptom* (Hillsdale, N.J.: The Analytic Press, 1991).

Blumenfeld, L. *The Big Book of Relaxation* (Rosyln, N.Y.: The Relaxation Company, 1994).

Bradshaw, J. *Bradshaw On: The Family* (Deerfield Beach, Fla.: Health Communications, Inc., 1988).

Brenner, C. *An Elementary Textbook of Psychoanalysis* (New York: Anchor Books, 1955).

Brown, S. *Treating the Alcoholic, A Developmental Approach* (New York: John Wiley and Sons, 1985).

Burns, D. D. *Feeling Good, The New Mood Therapy* (New York: Signet Books, 1980).

Chopra, D. *Ageless Body, Timeless Mind* (New York: Harmony Books, 1993).

Crisman, W. H. *The Opposite of Everything is True* (New York: Quill/William Morrow, 1991).

Ellis, A. *Anger—How to Live With It, and Without It* (N.J.: Citadel Press, 1977).

Fraiburg, S. H. *The Magic Years, Understanding and Handling the Problems of Early Childhood* (New York: Charles Scribner's Sons, 1959).

Frank, J. *Persuasion and Healing, A Comparative Study of Psychotherapy* (New York: Schocken Books, 1963).

Frankl, V. E. *Man's Search for Meaning* (New York: Simon and Schuster, 1959).

Freud, S. *Introductory Lectures on Psychoanalysis* (New York: W. W. Norton, 1966).

————. *The Complete Psychological Works of Sigmund Freud,* Edited and translated by J. Strachey, vol. 7 (London: Hogarth Press and Institute of Psychoanalysis, 1953), p. 289.

Friday, N. *My Mother/My Self, The Daughter's Search for Identity* (New York: Dell Publishing Co., 1977).

Fromm-Reichman, F. *Principles of Intensive Psychotherapy* (Chicago: University of Chicago Press, 1950).

Gabbard, K., and G. O. Jabbered. *Psychiatry and the Cinema* (Chicago: University of Chicago Press, 1987).

Geller, J. D., and P. D. Spector. *Psychotherapy, Portraits in Fiction* (Northvale, N.J.: Jason Aranson, Inc., 1987).

Goldberg, C. *On Being A Psychotherapist* (Northvale, N.J.: Jason Aranson, Inc., 1991).

Gravits, H. L., and J. D. Bowden. *Recovery, A Guide for Adult Children of Alcoholics* (New York: Simon and Schuster, Inc., 1985).

Harris, T. A. *I'm O.K., You're O.K.* (New York: HarperRow, 1948).

Hobson, R. F. *Forms of Feeling, The Heart of Psychotherapy* (New York: Tavistock Publications, 1985).

Isrealoff, R. *In Confidence: Four Years of Therapy* (Boston: Houghton Mifflin Co., 1990).

Kegan, R. *The Evolving Self, Problem and Process in Human Development* (Cambridge, Mass.: Harvard University Press, 1982).

Khantzian, E. J. "A contemporary psychodynamic approach to drug abuse treatment." Am. J. Drug Alcohol Abuse 12:213–222, 1986.

Lerner, H. G. *The Dance of Anger* (New York: HarperRow, 1985).

Luborsky, L., P. Crits-Christoph, J. Mintz, and A. Auerbach. *Who Will Benefit from Psychotherapy?* (New York: Basic Books, Inc., 1988).

Maslow, A. H. *The Farther Reaches of Human Nature* (New York: Penguin Books, 1971).

Mellody, P. *Facing Codependence* (San Francisco: HarperRow Publishers, 1988).

Miller, A. *Pictures of A Childhood* (New York: Farrar, Straus, and Giroux, 1986).

Peele, S. *Diseasing of America, Addiction Treatment Out of Control* (Boston: Houghton Mifflin, 1989).

Peele, S., and A. Brodsky. *The Truth About Addiction and Recovery* (New York: Simon Schuster, 1992).

Pope, K. S., and J. C. Bouhoutsos. *Sexual Intimacy Between Therapists and Patients* (New York: Preager, 1986).

Rippere, V., and R. Williams. *Wounded Healers, Mental Health Workers Experiences of Depression* (New York: John Wiley and Sons, 1985).

Robinson, N. *Getting Better, Inside Alcoholics Anonymous* (New York: William Morrow and Co., 1988).

Rogers, C. R. *A Way of Being* (Boston: Houghton Mifflin, Co., 1980).

Sacks, O. *The Man Who Mistook His Wife for a Hat and Other Clinical Tales* (New York: Harper and Row, 1970).

Seligman, M. P. *Helplessness* (San Francisco: W. H. Freeman and Co., 1975).

Sheehy, G. *Passages* (New York: Bantam, 1976).

Shem, S. *Fine* (New York: Dell Publishing, 1985).

Silverman, I. *Pure Types are Rare, Myths and Meanings of Madness* (New York: Praeger, 1983).

Stuart, G. W., and S. J. Sundeen. *Principles and Practice of Psychiatric Nursing*, 5th ed. (St. Louis: Mosby, 1995).

Sullivan, H. S. *Conceptions of Modern Psychiatry* (New York: W. W. Norton, 1940).

———. *Personal Psychopathology* (New York: W. W. Norton, 1972).

Sundberg, N. D., J. R. Taplin, and L. E. Tyler. *Introduction to Clinical Psychology* (Englewood Cliffs, N.J.: Prentice Hall, 1983).

Sussman, M. B. *A Curious Calling, Unconscious Motivations for Practicing Psychotherapy* (Northvale, N.J.: Jason Aranson Inc., 1992).

Weinberg, G. *The Heart of Psychotherapy* (New York: St. Martins Press, 1984).

Weiss, B. L. *Many Lives, Many Masters* (New York: Fireside Books, 1988).

Wilson, R. R. *Don't Panic, Taking Control of Anxiety Attacks* (New York: HarperRow, 1986).

Yalom, Irvin D., *Inpatient Group Psychotherapy.* (New York: Basic Books, Inc., 1983).

———. *Love's Executioner, and Other Tales of Psychotherapy* (New York: Basic Books, Inc., 1989).

Index